ALLE ZEIT WACH 1842

World Health Organization

The series *International Histological Classification of Tumours* consists of the following volumes. Each of these volumes – apart from volumes 1 and 2, which have already been revised – will appear in a revised edition within the next few years. Volumes of the current editions can be ordered through WHO, Distribution and Sales, Avenue Appia, CH-1211 Geneva 27.

1. Histological typing of lung tumours (1967, second edition 1981)
2. Histological typing of breast tumours (1968, second edition 1981)
3. Histological typing of soft tissue tumours (1969)
4. Histological typing of oral and oropharyngeal tumours (1971)
6. Histological typing of bone tumours (1972)
8. Cytology of the female genital tract (1973)
9. Histological typing of ovarian tumours (1973)
10. Histological typing of urinary bladder tumours (1973)
12. Histological typing of skin tumours (1974)
13. Histological typing of female genital tract tumours (1975)
14. Histological and cytological typing of neoplastic diseases of haematopoietic and lymphoid tissues (1976)
16. Histological typing of testis tumours (1977)
17. Cytology of non-gynaecological sites (1977)
20. Histological typing of tumours of the liver, biliary tract and pancreas (1978)
21. Histological typing of tumours of the central nervous system (1979)
22. Histological typing of prostate tumours (1980)
23. Histological typing of endocrine tumours (1980)
24. Histological typing of tumours of the eye and its adnexa (1980)
25. Histological typing of kidney tumours (1981)

A coded compendium of the International Histological Classification of Tumours (1978).

*The following volumes have already appeared in a revised edition with Springer Verlag:*
Histological Typing of Thyroid Tumours, 2nd edn. Hedinger/Williams/Sobin (1988)
Histological Typing of Intestinal Tumours, 2nd edn. Jass/Sobin (1989)
Histological Typing of Oesophageal and Gastric Tumours, 2nd edn. Watanabe/Jass/Sobin (1990)
Histological Typing of Tumours of the Gallbladder and Extrahepatic Bile Ducts, 2nd edn. Albores-Saavedra/Henson/Sobin (1990)
Histological Typing of Tumours of the Upper Respiratory Tract and Ear, 2nd edn. Shanmugaratnam/Sobin (1991)
Histological Typing of Salivary Gland Tumours, 2nd edn. Seifert (1991)
Histological Typing of Odontogenic Tumours, 2nd edn. Kramer/Pindborg/Shear (1992)

A set of 159 slides (121 in colour, 38 in monochrome), corresponding to the illustrations in the book, is available from the American Registry of Pathology, 14th Street and Alaska Ave. NW, Washington, DC 20306, USA. For further information please see p. 119.

# Histological Typing of Odontogenic Tumours

I. R. H. Kramer, J. J. Pindborg,
and M. Shear

Second Edition

With 142 Figures

Springer-Verlag Berlin Heidelberg GmbH

I. R. H. Kramer
Emeritus Professor of Oral Pathology, University of London, England

J. J. Pindborg
Professor of Oral Pathology, Royal Dental College, Copenhagen, Denmark
(WHO Collaborating Centre for the Histological Classification
of Odontogenic Tumours)

M. Shear
Deputy Vice-Chancellor and Honorary Professor of Oral Pathology
University of the Witwatersrand, Johannesburg, South Africa

In this series, colour illustrations will be limited in number in order to maintain a reasonable sales price.

In the present volume, we are greatly indebted to a number of donors, including the International Association of Oral Pathologists and Kodak Limited, whose generous contributions have made it possible for all of the photomicrographs to be reproduced in colour.

First edition published by WHO in 1971 as No. 5 in the International Histological Classification of Tumours series

ISBN 978-3-540-54142-4

Library of Congress Cataloging-in-Publication Data
Kramer, Ivor R. H. (Ivor Robert Horton) Histological typing of odontogenic tumours / I. R. H. Kramer, J. J. Pindborg, and M. Shear. – 2nd ed. p. cm. – (International histological classification of tumours) Rev. ed. of: Histological typing of odontogenic tumours, jaw cysts, and allied lesions / J. J. Pindborg, I. R. H. Kramer, in collaboration with H. Torloni, 1971. Includes index.
ISBN 978-3-540-54142-4 ISBN 978-3-662-02858-2 (eBook)
DOI 10.1007/978-3-662-02858-2
1. Odontogenic tumors–Histopathology. 2. Odontogenic tumors–Classification. I. Pindborg, J. J. (Jens Jorgen), 1921–Histological typing of odontogenic tumours, jaw cysts, and allied lesions. II. Pindborg, J. J. (Jens Jorgen), 1921– . III. Shear, Mervyn. IV. Title. V. Series: International histological classification of tumours (Unnumbered). [DNLM: 1. Odontogenic Tumors–classification. 2. Odontogenic Tumors–pathology. WU 280 K89h]
RC280.M6K73 1991 616.99'292-dc20 DNLM/DLC for Library of Congress 91-4996 CIP


Originally published by Springer-Verlag Berlin Heidelberg New York in 1992



Reproduction of the figures: Gustav Dreher GmbH, Stuttgart
Typesetting: Appl, Wemding;
24/3111-5 – Printed on acid-free paper
SPIN: 10757780

**Consultants**

*Abrams, A., Dr.*
Department of Oral Pathology, University of Southern California, Los Angeles, USA

*Buchner, A., Dr.*
Department of Oral Pathology, School of Dental Medicine, University of Tel Aviv, Israel

*Donath, K., Dr.*
Institute of Pathology, University of Hamburg, Germany

*Esguep, A., Dr.*
Department of Oral Pathology, Faculty of Odontology, University of Chile, Chile

*Hansen, L., Dr.*
Department of Oral Medicine and Hospital Dentistry, University of California, San Francisco, USA

*Nikai, H., Dr.*
Department of Oral Pathology, Hiroshima University, Japan

*Radden, B., Dr.*
Department of Dental Medicine and Surgery, University of Melbourne, Australia

**Reviewers**

*Rick, G., Dr.*
Oral Pathology Service, La Jolla, California, USA

*Lee, K. W., Dr.*
Department of Oral Pathology, Institute of Dental Surgery, University of London, England

*van der Waal, I., Dr.*
Department of Oral Pathology, Academic Hospital, Free University, Amsterdam, Netherlands

# General Preface to the Series

Among the prerequisites for comparative studies of cancer are international agreement on histological criteria for the definition and classification of cancer types and a standardized nomenclature. An internationally agreed classification of tumours, acceptable alike to physicians, surgeons, radiologists, pathologists and statisticians, would enable cancer workers in all parts of the world to compare their findings and would facilitate collaboration among them.

In a report published in 1952,[1] a subcommittee of the World Health Organization (WHO) Expert Committee on Health Statistics discussed the general principles that should govern the statistical classification of tumours and agreed that, to ensure the necessary flexibility and ease of coding, three separate classifications were needed according to (1) anatomical site, (2) histological type, and (3) degree of malignancy. A classification according to anatomical site is available in the International Classification of Diseases.[2]

In 1956, the WHO Executive Board passed a resolution[3] requesting the Director-General to explore the possibility that WHO might organize centres in various parts of the world and arrange for the collection of human tissues and their histological classification. The main purpose of such centres would be to develop histological definitions of cancer types and to facilitate the wide adoption of a uniform nomenclature. The resolution was endorsed by the Tenth World Health Assembly in May 1957.[4]

---

[1] WHO (1952) WHO Technical Report Series. No.53, 1952, p45

[2] WHO (1977) Manual of the international statistical classification of diseases, injuries, and causes of death. 1975 version. Geneva

[3] WHO (1956) WHO Official Records. No.68, p14 (resolution EB 17.R40)

[4] WHO (1957) WHO Official Records. No.79, p467 (resolution WHA 10.18)

Since 1958, WHO has established a number of centres concerned with this subject. The result of this endeavour has been the International Histological Classification of Tumours, a multivolumed series whose first edition was published between 1967 and 1981. The present revised second edition aims to update the classification, reflecting progress in diagnosis and the relevance of tumour types to clinical and epidemiological features.

# Preface to the Histological Typing of Odontogenic Tumours, Second Edition

The first edition of this book, entitled *Histological Typing of Odontogenic Tumours, Jaw Cysts and Allied Lesions,*[1] was the result of a collaborative effort organized by WHO and carried out by the International Reference Centre at the Department of Oral Pathology, Royal Dental College, Copenhagen, Denmark.

In order to keep the classification up to date, and in preparation for this new edition, the text of the first edition was circulated to the international panel of consultants listed on page V for their comments and suggestions. These, together with advice received from many other oral pathologists, were taken into account in the preparation of a new draft. After further preparatory work and discussion, a revised draft was sent to the three reviewers listed on page V, and their detailed comments were of the greatest help in the preparation of the final text. The authors would like to express their sincere appreciation of the help so freely given by the consultants and reviewers.

In this second edition the title has been modified for the sake of uniformity with other volumes in this series; the scope remains essentially the same as that of the first edition.

The histological classification which appears on pages 7–9 contains the morphology code numbers of the International Classification of Diseases for Oncology (ICD-O)[2] and the Systematized Nomenclature of Medicine (SNOMED).[3]

---

[1] Pindborg JJ, Kramer IRH (1971) Histological Typing of Odontogenic Tumours, Jaw Cysts, and Allied Lesions. Geneva, World Health Organization (International Histological Classification of Tumours, No. 5)

[2] World Health Organization (1990) International Classification of Diseases for Oncology. Geneva

[3] College of American Pathologists (1982) Systematized Nomenclature of Medicine. Chicago

It will, of course, be appreciated that the classification reflects the present state of knowledge, and modifications are almost certain to be needed as experience accumulates. Furthermore, the classification necessarily represents a majority view, from which some pathologists may wish to dissent. It is nevertheless hoped that, in the interests of international cooperation, all pathologists will use the classification as put forward. Criticisms and suggestions for its improvement will be welcomed; these should be sent to the World Health Organization, Geneva, Switzerland.

The publications in the series *International Histological Classification of Tumours* are not intended to serve as textbooks but rather to facilitate the adoption of a uniform terminology that will facilitate and improve communication among cancer workers. For this reason literature references have been omitted and readers should refer to standard works for bibliographies.

# Contents

# Introduction

## Inter-relationships of the Dental Tissues

The tooth germ has three main components – the enamel organ, the dental papilla and the dental follicle (Fig. 1). The enamel organ is an epithelial structure derived from the ectoderm that lines much of the oral cavity. The dental papilla and the dental follicle are ectomesenchymal (mesectodermal), being partly derived from cells that migrated from the neural crest early in embryogenesis. Both the gross morphology of the tooth germ and the differentiation of its cells depend upon a complex pattern of inductive interactions between the epithelium and the ectomesenchyme.

The sites in which the teeth will form appear to be determined before the commencement of epithelial downgrowth from the oral epithelium to form the odontogenic epithelium. This epithelial downgrowth (the dental lamina), the development of the enamel organs of the individual teeth, and the morphology of each enamel organ, are controlled by the ectomesenchyme.

The enamel organ is responsible for the formation of enamel and comprises four layers: outer dental epithelium, stellate reticulum, stratum intermedium and inner dental epithelium (Figs. 1 and 2a).

The dental papilla (Fig. 2b) is responsible for the formation of the dentine, and contact with epithelium provides the inductive stimulus necessary for the differentiation of odontoblasts on the surface of the papilla. When dentine formation starts (Fig. 3), this in turn provides the stimulus for the maturation of inner dental epithelial cells into functional ameloblasts and enamel is deposited on the dentine surface in the crown area. Later, a further extension from each enamel organ provides the epithelium necessary for the induction of odontoblast differentiation and dentine formation in the root area. The epithelial extension from the enamel organ breaks up, and residues (the epithelial rests of Malassez) persist throughout life in the periodontal ligament close to the root surface of each tooth. In the formed tooth, the dental papilla remains as the dental pulp, with the layer of odontoblasts at the periphery (Fig. 4).

The morphological and inductive relationships between the various parts of the normal tooth germ are reproduced, to a greater or lesser extent, in many of the tumours and tumour-like lesions of the odontogenic tissues. Thus, the observation of these features is important both in the identification of the lesions and in their classification.

For example, normal dentine is easily identified because of its tubular structure, but if for some reason this tubular structure is absent it is difficult to distinguish between atypical poorly mineralized dentine (dentinoid) and atypical osteoid. However, if an osteoid-like tissue develops in direct relationship to odontogenic epithelium, this relationship provides strong presumptive evidence that the material is, in fact, dysplastic dentine.

Cementum, which normally covers the dentine of the root of the tooth, exists in both acellular and cellular forms. Cementum is essentially a type of bundle bone, and both the cementum of the tooth and the bundle bone lining the tooth socket are produced by cells derived from the dental follicle. Cementum, especially the acellular variety, tends to exhibit a characteristic intense basophilia (Fig. 5). However, when cementum is deposited other than in its normal location on the root of a tooth, it may be difficult to distinguish from bone (see below).

Cementum and dentine, like bone, have a substantial collagenous matrix. The organic component of enamel is non-collagenous and is present in such small amounts that, when a specimen is demineralized before sectioning, the tenuous matrix of the enamel may be lost. However, in some circumstances (especially when enamel is enclosed by other tissues) the matrix may be retained (Fig. 6). Globules of basophilic mineralized material in contact with ameloblastic epithelium may represent dysplastic enamel.

## Cementum-Containing Lesions

Within the normal periodontal ligament, next to the cementum covering the root of the tooth and sometimes fused to the cementum, it is not uncommon to find occasional rounded, strongly basophilic calcified masses. In this location it is reasonable to suppose that these masses are derived from the type of cell that forms the adjacent cementum, and they are termed 'cementicles'. When similar masses are found in certain tumours and tumour-like lesions of the jaws, often fused into larger aggregates and sometimes intermingled with deposits of bone, it is reasonable again to regard them as a form of cementum; this supposition is reflected in the names by which these lesions are known (eg. 'cementifying fibroma', 'cemento-ossifying fibroma').

However, it must be recognized that similar cementum-like material may be found in lesions of parts of the craniofacial skeleton other than the jaws, and occasionally in other parts of the skeleton – locations in which it is not possible to envisage derivation from the odontogenic tissues. These observations may be attributable to the fact that, although formed by cells of the odontogenic apparatus, cementum is a form of bundle bone. Therefore, it is understandable that sometimes tissue of similar appearance may be found in locations other than the jaws.

The classification of odontogenic tumours has to include provision for lesions in which there is hard tissue that may be cementum, or bone, or a mixture of the two – lesions which might be described under the heading 'Neoplasms and other tumours related to the odontogenic apparatus' or in the category of 'Neoplasms and other lesions related to bone'. In this revision, the one neoplasm that is generally accepted as being essentially cementogenic (the benign cementoblastoma) has been included in the former category, whilst the cemento-ossifying lesions (both neoplastic and dysplastic) are listed in the category of 'Neoplasms and other lesions related to bone'.

## Scope of the Classification

The primary purpose of the following classification is to list and define neoplasms, tumour-like lesions and cysts arising from the odontogenic apparatus. However, the classification also includes some distinctive jaw lesions that are of uncertain status, and others that are clearly non-neoplastic but must be distinguished from odontogenic neoplasms. The classification includes a few types of odontogenic tumours that have been described quite recently, so that only a preliminary picture is available of their clinical and histopathological characteristics. It is hoped that including reference to them here will make possible the identification and description of further cases, so that a more detailed knowledge of their characteristics can be achieved.

Types of bone tumour that also occur in other parts of the skeleton and do not show special features when occurring in the jaws are not included, although certain bone tumours and tumour-like lesions that are distinctive when occurring in the jaws are discussed.

Similarly, soft tissue tumours that are not peculiar to the jaws but may occur within the jaws are not considered, unless they present special problems in differential diagnosis. Metastatic deposits in the jaws are also excluded.

Other volumes in this series that will be helpful in the identification of tumours of the orofacial region include –

Soft Tissue Tumours
Oral and Oropharyngeal Tumours
Bone Tumours
Salivary Gland Tumours

## Classification of Odontogenic Tumours

Over the years there have been many attempts to produce a 'logical' classification of tumours and tumour-like lesions of the odontogenic tissues. Recent advances in our understanding of the origins and the interactions of these tissues have provided a sounder scientific basis for classification, but uncertainties remain, partly because of the complexity of the tissues involved and partly because the rarity of some lesions makes it difficult to accumulate a large series for study and comparison.

The classification used here is based firstly on tumour behaviour, with a broad division into lesions generally regarded as 'benign' and those regarded as 'malignant'; the 'benign' category includes a number of entities that are probably or certainly non-neoplastic. Subdivisions of the 'benign' lesions are then based on the types of odontogenic tissues involved: odontogenic epithelium without odontogenic ectomesenchyme; odontogenic epithelium with odontogenic ectomesenchyme; odontogenic ectomesenchyme with or without included odontogenic epithelium. The word 'included' in the latter group is intended to indicate that, although epithelium may be present, it sometimes appears to be included by chance rather than playing any essential role in the pathogenesis of the lesion.

Lesions made up of odontogenic epithelium with odontogenic ectomesenchyme have the elements necessary for inductive interactions leading to the formation of dentine and then enamel. Whether or not these dental hard tissues are found in any individual case depends in part on the stage at which the lesion is excised, and in part on factors that are not yet understood. It is possible that some of the lesions given separate designations in the present classification are simply chronological stages in the evolution of a single type of tumour; until larger numbers of examples have been studied, it is suggested that they should be placed into the separate categories provided, so that differences in presentation and behaviour may be more easily assessed.

## Notes on Terminology

1. Where there is good evidence that a lesion is neoplastic, this will be stated in the brief definition of the lesion that precedes the detailed description.
2. Where there is good evidence that a lesion represents a developmental anomaly or malformation, this will also be stated in the brief definition.
3. In accordance with common practice, the terms 'lesion' and 'lesional tissue' will be used for both neoplastic and non-neoplastic disorders.
4. Synonyms are given where they have been widely used in the literature; the preferred term is given first, followed by the synonym in brackets.

# Histological Classification of Odontogenic Tumours

| | | |
|---|---|---|
| 1 | **Neoplasms and Other Tumours Related to the Odontogenic Apparatus** | |
| 1.1 | **Benign** | |
| 1.1.1 | *Odontogenic epithelium without odontogenic ectomesenchyme* | |
| 1.1.1.1 | Ameloblastoma | 9310/0[a] |
| 1.1.1.2 | Squamous odontogenic tumour | 9312/0 |
| 1.1.1.3 | Calcifying epithelial odontogenic tumour (Pindborg tumour) | 9340/0 |
| 1.1.1.4 | Clear cell odontogenic tumour | 9270/0 |
| 1.1.2 | *Odontogenic epithelium with odontogenic ectomesenchyme, with or without dental hard tissue formation* | |
| 1.1.2.1 | Ameloblastic fibroma | 9330/0 |
| 1.1.2.2 | Ameloblastic fibrodentinoma (dentinoma) and ameloblastic fibro-odontoma | 9290/0 |
| 1.1.2.3 | Odontoameloblastoma | 9311/0 |
| 1.1.2.4 | Adenomatoid odontogenic tumour | 9300/0 |
| 1.1.2.5 | Calcifying odontogenic cyst | 9301/0 |
| 1.1.2.6 | Complex odontoma | 9282/0 |
| 1.1.2.7 | Compound odontoma | 9281/0 |
| 1.1.3 | *Odontogenic ectomesenchyme with or without included odontogenic epithelium* | |
| 1.1.3.1 | Odontogenic fibroma | See note 1 |
| 1.1.3.2 | Myxoma (odontogenic myxoma, myxofibroma) | 9320/0 |
| 1.1.3.3 | Benign cementoblastoma (cementoblastoma, true cementoma) | 9273/0 |

[a] Morphology code of the International Classification of Diseases for Oncology (ICD-O) and the Systematized Nomenclature of Medicine (SNOMED)

[1] Central odontogenic fibroma 9321/0, peripheral odontogenic fibroma 9322/0

## 1.2 Malignant

| | | |
|---|---|---|
| 1.2.1 | *Odontogenic carcinomas* | |
| 1.2.1.1 | Malignant ameloblastoma | 9310/3 |
| 1.2.1.2 | Primary intraosseous carcinoma | 9270/3 |
| 1.2.1.3 | Malignant variants of other odontogenic epithelial tumours | See note 2 |
| 1.2.1.4 | Malignant changes in odontogenic cysts | 9270/3 |
| 1.2.2 | *Odontogenic sarcomas* | |
| 1.2.2.1 | Ameloblastic fibrosarcoma (ameloblastic sarcoma) | 9330/3 |
| 1.2.2.2 | Ameloblastic fibrodentinosarcoma and ameloblastic fibro-odontosarcoma | 9290/3 |
| 1.2.3 | Odontogenic carcinosarcoma | 8980/3 |

# 2 Neoplasms and Other Lesions Related to Bone

| | | |
|---|---|---|
| 2.1. | **Osteogenic neoplasms** | |
| 2.1.1 | Cemento-ossifying fibroma (cementifying fibroma, ossifying fibroma) | See note 3 |
| 2.2 | **Non-neoplastic bone lesions** | |
| 2.2.1 | Fibrous dysplasia of the jaws | 74910 |
| 2.2.2 | *Cemento-osseous dysplasias* | |
| 2.2.2.1 | Periapical cemental dysplasia (periapical fibrous dysplasia) | 9272/0 |
| 2.2.2.2 | Florid cemento-osseous dysplasia (gigantiform cementoma, familial multiple cementomas) | 9275/0 |
| 2.2.2.3 | Other cemento-osseous dysplasias | |
| 2.2.3 | Cherubism (familial multilocular cystic disease of the jaws) | 70980 |
| 2.2.4 | Central giant cell granuloma | 44130 |
| 2.2.5 | Aneurysmal bone cyst | 33640 |
| 2.2.6 | Solitary bone cyst (traumatic, simple, haemorrhagic bone cyst) | 33404 |

[2] Use appropriate tumour coding from 1.1 above, with behaviour code /3.

[3] Ossifying fibroma 9262/0, cementifying fibroma 9274/0.
9262/0 is recommended for cemento-ossifying fibroma.

| | | |
|---|---|---|
| 2.3 | **Other tumours** | |
| 2.3.1 | Melanotic neuroectodermal tumour of infancy (melanotic progonoma) . . . . . . . . . . . . . . . . | 9363/0 |

## 3 Epithelial Cysts

| | | |
|---|---|---|
| 3.1 | **Developmental** | |
| 3.1.1 | *Odontogenic* | |
| 3.1.1.1 | "Gingival cysts" of infants (Epstein pearls) . . . . | 26540 |
| 3.1.1.2 | Odontogenic keratocyst (primordial cyst) . . . . . | 26530 |
| 3.1.1.3 | Dentigerous (follicular) cyst . . . . . . . . . . . . . | 26560 |
| 3.1.1.4 | Eruption cyst . . . . . . . . . . . . . . . . . . . . . . . | 26550 |
| 3.1.1.5 | Lateral periodontal cyst . . . . . . . . . . . . . . . . | 26520 |
| 3.1.1.6 | Gingival cyst of adults . . . . . . . . . . . . . . . . . | 26540 |
| 3.1.1.7 | Glandular odontogenic cyst; sialo-odontogenic cyst | 26520 |
| 3.1.2 | *Non-odontogenic* | |
| 3.1.2.1 | Nasopalatine duct (incisive canal) cyst . . . . . . . | 26600 |
| 3.1.2.2 | Nasolabial (nasoalveolar) cyst . . . . . . . . . . . . | 26500 |

| | | |
|---|---|---|
| 3.2 | **Inflammatory** | |
| 3.2.1 | Radicular cyst . . . . . . . . . . . . . . . . . . . . . . | 43800 |
| 3.2.1.1 | Apical and lateral | |
| 3.2.1.2 | Residual | |
| 3.2.2 | Paradental (inflammatory collateral, mandibular infected buccal) cyst . . . . . . . . . . | 26520 |

# Definitions and Explanatory Notes

## 1 Neoplasms and Other Tumours Related to the Odontogenic Apparatus

## 1.1 Benign

### 1.1.1 Odontogenic Epithelium without Odontogenic Ectomesenchyme

#### 1.1.1.1 Ameloblastoma

*A benign but locally invasive polymorphic neoplasm consisting of proliferating odontogenic epithelium, which usually has a follicular or plexiform pattern, lying in a fibrous stroma.*

Most ameloblastomas occur as intraosseous growths arising from remnants of odontogenic epithelium, although as they enlarge there may be secondary fusion with the oral epithelium.

Usually the ameloblastomas are diagnosed in the 4th and 5th decades of life, except the unicystic variety, which is usually found in the 2nd and 3rd decades.

Over 80% of ameloblastomas occur in the mandible and the remainder in the maxilla. In the mandible, about 70% are in the molar region and the ascending ramus, 20% in the premolar region, and 10% in the incisor region.

Radiographically, the ameloblastoma may show considerable variation. The typical picture is of a multilocular destruction of bone (Fig. 7), but unilocular ameloblastomas also occur. Embedded teeth may be present in a variety of relationships to the tumour.

Histologically, the ameloblastoma occurs in two main patterns: *follicular* and *plexiform*. However, not infrequently both patterns are present in the same tumour.

In the *follicular* pattern (Fig. 8) the tumour epithelium is in the form of more or less discrete islands. These consist of a central mass of polyhedral cells, or loosely connected angular cells resembling stellate reticulum, surrounded by a layer of cuboidal or columnar cells resembling internal dental epithelium or preameloblasts. Commonly, cysts form within the epithelial islands (Fig. 9).

In the *plexiform* pattern (Fig. 10) the tumour epithelium is arranged as a network which is bounded by a layer of cuboidal to columnar cells and includes cells resembling stellate reticulum. The latter are often less numerous than in the follicular type. Cyst formation occurs but is usually due to stromal degeneration rather than to a cystic change within the epithelium.

**Unicystic Ameloblastoma.** Three histological variants of the unicystic ameloblastoma have been described. In the first, a relatively innocuous epithelial lining may, in parts, show transformation to one with cuboidal or columnar basal cells with hyperchromatic nuclei, nuclear palisading with polarization, cytoplasmic vacuolization with intercellular spacing, and subepithelial hyalinization. In the second variant the cyst lining is similar to that of the first (Fig. 11 a), but a localized nodule arises from part of this lining and projects into the lumen of the cyst. The nodule comprises odontogenic epithelium with a plexiform pattern resembling that seen in the plexiform ameloblastoma (Fig. 11 b). This variety is sometimes referred to as the *plexiform unicystic ameloblastoma.* In the third variety, sometimes referred to as *mural ameloblastoma,* some part of the wall of the cyst is infiltrated by typical plexiform or follicular ameloblastoma. Sectioning at many levels is essential to ascertain the presence of mural involvement.

The first and second variants appear to require nothing further than enucleation, whereas in the third variant there may be infiltration of adjacent bone as in other forms of ameloblastoma.

The diagnosis of unicystic ameloblastoma is made histologically, and cannot be predicted preoperatively on clinical or radiographic grounds.

Cellular variants of the two main patterns of ameloblastoma are:

a) *Acanthomatous* (Fig. 12). This term is applied when there is extensive squamous metaplasia, sometimes with keratin formation, within the islands of tumour cells. Usually the general pattern of the tumour is that of the follicular type. This variety must be distinguished from the squamous odontogenic tumour (page 14), in which the peripheral cells are flat rather than columnar.

b) *Granular cell type* (Fig. 13). Ameloblastomas sometimes show a granular transformation of groups of the epithelial cells. Occasionally, a tumour is seen in which almost all of the epithelium is of this type, and when the granular cell change is extensive the tumour is referred to as the granular cell type. The cells are large and may be cuboidal, columnar or rounded. Their bulky cytoplasm is filled with acidophilic granules, which resemble lysosomes ultrastructurally and histochemically.

It should be noted that, in a variety of other lesions which contain odontogenic epithelium, a granular change may be seen in some of the epithelial cells.

**Other Variations.** In any ameloblastoma, but especially in the follicular type, there may be marked hyalinization of the connective tissue adjacent to the epithelium (Fig. 14).

The stroma of ameloblastomas usually consists of relatively acellular loose connective tissue. Sometimes it is more collagenous, and may be frankly desmoplastic with small nests and strands of odontogenic epithelium. This has been described as the *desmoplastic ameloblastoma* (Fig. 15).

Rarely, an ameloblastoma may show a predominantly basaloid pattern (Fig. 16), and this type of tumour is sometimes referred to as a *basal cell ameloblastoma.* When a basal cell type of growth occurs in the jaws, special care is necessary to distinguish between this type of ameloblastoma and an intraosseous adenoid cystic carcinoma.

Sometimes an ameloblastoma will show a limited amount of dystrophic mineralization. This occurs within the epithelium and should be distinguished from the mineralized masses in the calcifying epithelial odontogenic tumour, and from the dental hard tissue formation in the adenomatoid odontogenic tumour and other lesions.

In most ameloblastomas keratinization is absent or limited. Occasionally there is more extensive keratinization *(keratoameloblastoma)* and in a very rare variant *(papilliferous keratoameloblastoma)* some microcysts are lined by parakeratinized epithelium and contain keratin, whilst others have a non-keratinized epithelium with a papilliferous pattern (Figs. 17, 18).

As indicated earlier, most ameloblastomas arise from intraosseous residues of odontogenic epithelium. However, some ameloblastomas *(peripheral ameloblastoma)* appear to arise directly from the surface epithelium or from residues of the dental lamina lying outside the bone (Fig. 19).

It is also generally agreed that ameloblastomas may also arise as a result of a neoplastic change in the wall of a non-neoplastic odontogenic cyst, but opinions differ regarding the proportion of tumours that arise in this way. Figure 20 illustrates the development of an ameloblastoma in a dentigerous cyst.

Although the above list of types, or variants, of ameloblastoma gives the main histological patterns that may be encountered, it should be noted that, with the exception of the unicystic and the peripheral lesions and the desmoplastic ameloblastoma, there appear to be no consistent variations in clinical behaviour associated with these patterns.

In general, these tumours tend to spread through the cancellous bone (Fig. 21). They may cause resorption of compact bone but do not infiltrate the Haversian canals.

Unicystic ameloblastomas, peripheral ameloblastomas and possibly desmoplastic ameloblastomas have lower recurrence rates than other ameloblastomas.

### 1.1.1.2 Squamous Odontogenic Tumour

*A benign but locally infiltrative neoplasm consisting of islands of well-differentiated squamous epithelium in a fibrous stroma. The epithelial islands occasionally show foci of central cystic degeneration.*

The squamous odontogenic tumour probably arises from residues or derivatives of the dental lamina or from the rests of Malassez.

The tumour has been found from the 2nd to the 7th decades of life, with most occurring in the 3rd. There is no sex predilection, the maxilla and mandible are equally affected, and in some instances the lesion is multicentric. Most cases have shown a unilocular radiolucency.

The main histological features are islands of well-differentiated squamous epithelium set in a mature connective tissue stroma (Fig. 22). These epithelial islands have a peripheral layer of flattened or cuboidal cells, and lack the columnar cells that are typical of the ameloblastoma. In about half of the cases there are microscopic foci of degeneration and/or calcified areas within the tumour islands.

Some of the cases have an aggressive clinical behaviour, but it appears that curettage is the treatment of choice, and there have been few recurrences.

### 1.1.1.3 Calcifying Epithelial Odontogenic Tumour (Pindborg Tumour)

*A locally invasive epithelial neoplasm characterized by the development of intraepithelial structures, probably of an amyloid-like nature, which may become calcified and which may be liberated as the cells break down.*

The calcifying epithelial odontogenic tumour has been found with approximately the same frequency in the 4 decades between the ages of 20 and 60 years. In two-thirds of the cases the mandible is affected and in one-third the maxilla.

The prevalence in the molar region is three times that in the premolar region, whereas in the other sites of the jaws there is a fairly even distribution. Among extraosseous cases there seems to be a predilection for the anterior region. Most of these tumours are intraosseous, and in about half of the cases the lesion has been associated with an unerupted or embedded tooth or teeth.

The calcifying epithelial odontogenic tumour most commonly presents as a painless mass that has been slowly enlarging.

The characteristic radiographic appearance is of an irregular radiolucent area, containing radiopaque masses of varying size which tend to be located close to the crown of the unerupted tooth (Fig. 23). At the periphery the radiolucent zone may or may not be clearly demarcated from the normal bone.

Histologically, the tumour shows a considerable variation. There are sheets or strands of polyhedral epithelial cells which have well-defined cell borders and which often show distinct intercellular bridges (Fig. 24), and a fibrous stroma that may show degenerative changes. There is usually pleomorphism of the tumour epithelium (Fig. 25); giant nuclei, multinucleated cells and cells with prominent nucleoli are often a feature of the epithelium, but mitoses are rarely seen. Variants showing a preponderance of clear cells have also been reported. Within the sheets of tumour cells are rounded, acidophilic, homogeneous masses which commonly calcify and may show Liesegang rings (Fig. 26), although in a few instances no calcifications are found. Special staining techniques, especially thioflavine T, show that the homogeneous material gives reactions similar to those of amyloid (Fig. 27).

There is some controversy as to the nature of the amyloid-like material: whether it is a degeneration product or is actively secreted. The surrounding epithelial cells may degenerate, with the result that the acidophilic and mineralized masses are liberated. The stroma may contain strongly basophilic bodies, which are irregular or angular and which sometimes fuse to form complex masses.

In the peripheral or extraosseous type the neoplastic epithelium appears to be less active (Fig. 28), and there are fewer foci of calcification than in the intraosseous type.

In a few tumours, part of the lesion has the pattern of the calcifying epithelial odontogenic tumour and part has the pattern of the adenomatoid odontogenic tumour.

#### 1.1.1.4 Clear Cell Odontogenic Tumour

*A benign but locally invasive neoplasm originating from odontogenic epithelium and characterized by sheets and islands of uniform, vacuolated and clear cells.*

This neoplasm has been described only recently and few cases have been published; it is therefore too early to give a comprehensive picture.

The clear cell odontogenic tumour probably arises from residues or derivatives of the dental lamina or from rests of Malassez. It occurs as a central tumour in either jaw, in the form of a radiolucent lesion often with poorly defined margins.

The main histological features are sheets, strands and islands of uniform vacuolated, clear or finely stippled cells without evidence of glandular differentiation (Fig. 29). Many tumour cells contain abundant glycogen granules. Ultrastructurally, many cells exhibit prominent vacuolization and a paucity of cytoplasmic organelles. The mature fibrous stroma is scanty, and there is no evidence of amyloid deposition or calcification.

The tumour has some similarity in appearance to clear cell adenocarcinoma. It seems to be more locally aggressive than ameloblastoma.

### 1.1.2 Odontogenic Epithelium With Odontogenic Ectomesenchyme, With or Without Dental Hard Tissue Formation

#### Ameloblastic Fibroma and Related Lesions

*Neoplasms composed of proliferating odontogenic epithelium embedded in a cellular ectomesenchymal tissue that resembles the dental papilla, and with varying degrees of inductive change and dental hard tissue formation.*

There is a variety of lesions that consists of a disorderly mixture of odontogenic epithelium and odontogenic ectomesenchyme. Some are developmental anomalies (see complex and compound odontomata): in their later stages these will show inductive changes and lay down increasing amounts of dental hard tissues until the growth of the lesion is completed. Other lesions, grouped here under the heading 'ameloblastic fibroma and related lesions', are benign neoplasms. All of these are rare, and until more experience has been gained it may be worthwhile separately identifying the differing patterns or types, even though some of these may later prove to be nothing more than stages in the evolution of a single type of tumour.

These neoplasms tend to occur in children. As developing odontomata are also usually found in children, special care is needed to distinguish such self-limiting developmental anomalies from the neoplasms described here.

### 1.1.2.1 Ameloblastic Fibroma

This tumour usually occurs in a much younger age group than does the ameloblastoma and is not commonly seen in individuals over 21 years of age.

Ameloblastic fibroma shows a well-defined cystic radiolucency, usually in the premolar-molar region of the mandible, and radiographic differentiation from ameloblastoma may be impossible.

The epithelial component is usually in the form of strands and islands, often consisting of a peripheral layer of cuboidal or columnar cells which may enclose a small number of cells resembling stellate reticulum (Fig. 30). Cyst formation within the epithelium is not common, and the cysts remain small. In some tumours the epithelial cells are mainly rounded or cuboidal and arranged in slender strands.

The connective tissue component is much more cellular than in ameloblastoma; the cells are rounded or angular, and there is little collagen (Fig. 31). There may be a narrow cell-free zone bordering the epithelium, and sometimes juxtaepithelial hyalinization of the type seen in the ordinary ameloblastoma. Occasionally the hyalinization is more diffuse.

In a few instances a variable proportion of the stromal cells exhibit a finely granular cytoplasm, and such tumours are sometimes termed *granular cell ameloblastic fibroma.*

There is evidence that both the epithelial and the connective tissue components of ameloblastic fibroma are neoplastic.

### 1.1.2.2 Ameloblastic Fibrodentinoma (Dentinoma) and Ameloblastic Fibro-odontoma

*Lesions similar to ameloblastic fibroma, but also showing inductive changes that lead to the formation of dentine, and, in ameloblastic fibro-odontoma, enamel as well.*

Radiographically, ameloblastic fibrodentinoma appears as a well-defined radiolucency containing varying amounts of radiopaque material.

The epithelium is usually in the form of slender strands consisting of no more than a double layer of rounded or cuboidal cells, and much of the connective tissue may resemble that of the dental papilla. In addition, a poorly organized dentine is deposited (Fig. 32); strands of the odontogenic epithelium are closely associated with this dentine and some may become incorporated. Usually the dentine is poorly mineralized, and it contains entrapped mesenchymal cells in addition to the entrapped epithelium. Relatively well-formed tubular dentine is a rare finding, but the margins of the masses of forming dentine often show radially arranged coarse fibre bundles with elongated cells lying between and parallel to the bundles (Fig. 32).

Most ameloblastic fibrodentinomas occur within bone, but a few lie outside, and occasionally the contained epithelium may have been derived directly from the oral mucosa.

Ameloblastic fibro-odontoma is similar to ameloblastic fibrodentinoma, with the same association of odontogenic epithelium and cell-rich mesenchyme, but here the inductive changes are further advanced and enamel is present in addition to dentine (Fig. 33).

The radiographic appearance, like that of ameloblastic fibrodentinoma, is of a well-defined radiolucency containing varying amounts of radiopaque material (Fig. 34). As in the case of the other lesions described in this section, distinction from a developing odontoma is important but may be difficult. In addition to the histological features, careful consideration must be given to the age of the patient and to the location of the lesion (for example, if it is directly overlying the crown of an unerupted tooth in a young subject, it is likely to be a developing odontoma rather than a neoplasm).

### 1.1.2.3 Odontoameloblastoma

*A very rare neoplasm which includes odontogenic ectomesenchyme, in addition to odontogenic epithelium that resembles an ameloblasto-*

*ma both in structure and in behaviour. Because of the presence of the odontogenic ectomesenchyme, inductive changes take place leading to the formation of dentine and enamel in parts of the tumour.*

Radiographically the tumour presents as a radiolucency similar to that of an ameloblastoma, but within which mineralized tissue can be detected. Histologically the tumour epithelium is typical of an ameloblastoma, but in addition to fibrous stroma there is a variable amount of typically cellular odontogenic ectomesenchyme (Fig. 35), and both dentine and enamel will be formed.

### 1.1.2.4 Adenomatoid Odontogenic Tumour

*A tumour of odontogenic epithelium with duct-like structures and with varying degrees of inductive change in the connective tissue. The tumour may be partly cystic, and in some cases the solid lesion may be present only as masses in the wall of a large cyst. It is generally believed that the lesion is not a neoplasm.*

The tumour is seen more frequently in female patients, it usually occurs in the 2nd decade of life, and presents as a slow-growing, painless swelling. The maxilla is involved nearly twice as frequently as the mandible, the anterior part of the maxilla, especially the canine region, being the most common site. The tumour is commonly associated with an unerupted tooth and may closely simulate a dentigerous cyst both radiographically (Fig. 36 a) and at operation, but in some cases the presence of calcified material within the adenomatoid odontogenic tumour may be a useful diagnostic feature (Fig. 36 b).

Histologically, the tumour may be solid or there may be more or less extensive cyst formation (Fig. 37). The epithelium is in the form of whorled masses of spindle cells as well as sheets and plexiform strands. Rings of columnar cells give rise to a duct-like appearance (Fig. 38), but such structures may be scanty. Between opposing rows of columnar cells there is often an acidophilic material that is usually periodic acid-Schiff (PAS) positive. Immunohistochemical studies have shown this to be basement membrane-like material.

The connective tissue component includes varying amounts of acidophilic hyaline material, often containing strands of entrapped epithelium. This hyaline material appears to be dysplastic dentine (Fig. 39), and occasionally a tubular pattern is seen in some areas. Very rarely the formation of enamel matrix has been observed, and amyloid-like material may also be present. Calcification is sometimes seen and may be extensive.

The adenomatoid odontogenic tumour is usually encapsulated and is readily enucleated.

#### 1.1.2.5 Calcifying Odontogenic Cyst

*A cystic lesion in which the epithelial lining shows a well-defined basal layer of columnar cells, an overlying layer that is often many cells thick and that may resemble stellate reticulum, and masses of 'ghost' epithelial cells that may be in the epithelial cyst lining or in the fibrous capsule. The 'ghost' epithelial cells may become calcified. Dysplastic dentine may be laid down adjacent to the basal layer of the epithelium, and in some instances the cyst is associated with an area of more extensive dental hard tissue formation resembling that of a complex or compound odontoma.*

The lesion is most commonly found in the 2nd decade of life, with an almost equal sex distribution and a similar incidence in the mandible and the maxilla.

Radiographically, the lesion appears as a well-defined radiolucency containing varying amounts of radiopaque material (Fig. 40).

Calcifying odontogenic cyst usually occurs within bone but may also occur in the soft tissues of the tooth-bearing area.

Parts of the lesion often bear a striking resemblance to an ameloblastoma (Fig. 41) and previously most cases were diagnosed as atypical ameloblastomas. 'Ghost' epithelial cells (Figs. 41, 42), often calcified like those seen in pilomatrixoma, are one of the most distinctive features of the calcifying odontogenic cyst, although such cells may also occur in the ameloblastoma and in certain other odontogenic epithelial lesions.

Various stains, e.g. Goldner stain, van Gieson, and fluorescence microscopy after staining with rhodamine B (Fig. 43), may be useful in distinguishing between the ghost cells and other acidophilic masses. The staining reaction of the ghost cells suggests that they are keratinizing, and they are entirely thioflavine T-negative.

The cyst wall shows areas with more or less extensive proliferation, which may extend into the cyst cavity. As indicated earlier, dental hard tissue formation may be minimal or extensive (Fig. 44).

Most lesions with the features described above appear to be non-neoplastic. An exception is when the lesion also has ameloblastoma-like areas. Such tumours may have an infiltrative pattern of growth. The terms *dentinogenic ghost cell tumour* or *odontogenic ghost cell tumour* have been proposed for a predominantly solid lesion with features of ameloblastoma, ghost cells and dentinoid. This tumour usually occurs in older patients.

There is a rare variant of calcifying odontogenic cyst in which melanin forms in the epithelium.

### 1.1.2.6 Complex Odontoma

*A malformation in which all the dental tissues are represented, individual tissues being mainly well formed but occurring in a more or less disorderly pattern.*

The lesion occurs most commonly in the premolar or molar region. The active growth phase is during the formation of the dentition, and those lesions that cause expansion of the bone are usually diagnosed during the first 2 decades of life. Smaller lesions may be an incidental radiographic finding in adults.

Radiographically, the lesion commences as a well-defined radiolucency in which there is progressive deposition of radiopaque material of a nodular nature (Fig. 45).

Although complex odontoma consists primarily of a disordered mixture of dental tissues (Fig. 46), some examples include better-ordered, tooth-like structures. As already mentioned, during its development complex odontoma may be difficult to distinguish from ameloblastic fibroma or fibro-odontoma, and even when growth has been completed, residues of the odontogenic epithelium may still be identifiable (Fig. 47). Although the growth is self-limiting, the lesion may recur if it is incompletely removed at its early, predominantly soft tissue, stage.

### 1.1.2.7 Compound Odontoma

*A malformation in which all the dental tissues are represented in a more orderly pattern than in the complex odontoma, so that the lesion consists of many tooth-like structures. Most of these structures do not morphologically resemble the teeth of the normal dentition, but in each one enamel, dentine, cementum and pulp are arranged as in the normal tooth.*

The distinction between compound and complex odontomas is arbitrary, being based on a preponderance of well-organized denticles as against a preponderance of disorganized dental tissues rather than on any absolute difference. An example of the radiographic appearance is shown in Fig. 48 a, and Fig. 48 b shows the contents of the same lesion separated into its individual denticles.

## 1.1.3 Odontogenic Ectomesenchyme With or Without Included Odontogenic Epithelium

### 1.1.3.1 Odontogenic Fibroma

*A fibroblastic neoplasm containing varying amounts of apparently inactive odontogenic epithelium.*

This neoplasm is relatively rare and controversy exists as to the concept and the definition. At present the term 'odontogenic fibroma' appears to be applied to various types of lesion. One resembles dental follicle both in location and in structure; tissue of this type is referred to later under the heading "Myxoma".

Another and less common lesion is composed of a more cellular fibrous tissue, containing islands and strands of odontogenic epithelium (Fig. 49). However, the epithelial component may be so abundant that it is tempting to consider the lesion an epithelial tumour. This second type, which is usually encapsulated or sharply demarcated, may contain varying amounts of hard tissue resembling dysplastic cementum or bone (Fig. 50).

Occasionally, the fibrous component of an odontogenic fibroma will show variable numbers of cells with an acidophilic granular cytoplasm. The term *granular cell odontogenic tumour* is sometimes applied to tumours of this type, and to ameloblastic fibromas showing similar granular cells (see page 17).

Further subdivision of this group may become necessary, but at present criteria have not been agreed and differences in behaviour have not been established.

Not all central fibromas of the jaws contain epithelium, and in some the epithelial component is sparse. In the absence of epithelium, the diagnosis of odontogenic fibroma should be made with caution.

Extraosseous lesions exist *(peripheral odontogenic fibroma)* that have similar patterns to those described above. Sometimes the proliferation of odontogenic epithelium is so marked (Fig. 51) that it may be difficult to distinguish from a peripheral ameloblastoma.

There is also a distinctive gingival lesion, composed of strands and islands of epithelium in a mature fibrous stroma (Fig. 52), that rarely exceeds 1 cm in diameter and does not cause destruction of the underlying bone. This lesion appears to be non-neoplastic, and is known as *odontogenic gingival epithelial hamartoma.*

### 1.1.3.2 Myxoma (Odontogenic Myxoma, Myxofibroma)

*A locally invasive neoplasm consisting of rounded and angular cells lying in an abundant mucoid stroma.*

Radiographically, myxoma commonly shows multiple radiolucent areas of varying size (Fig. 53 a) separated by straight or curved bony septa ('soap-bubble' appearance). This picture may be indistinguishable from that of an ameloblastoma. It may also present as an ill-defined radiolucency.

Myxoma of the jaws is a tumour that shows little encapsulation. It often extends through the bone (Fig. 53 b) and into the soft tissues without any well-defined margin, so that complete removal is difficult and recurrences are common. Growth may be quite rapid and is probably due mainly to the accumulation of mucoid ground substance (Figs. 54, 55), as mitoses are rarely seen. Atypical nuclei (Fig. 56) are occasionally seen, but these tumours do not metastasize. Most odontogenic myxomas contain little collagen, but some contain a moderate amount, often in the form of isolated thick hyalinized bands. Depending upon the amount of collagen, some of these neoplasms are called myxofibromas. Scattered islands or strands of inactive-looking odontogenic epithelium, occasionally surrounded by a zone of hyalinization, may be found in some of the myxomas.

When a tooth fails to erupt, the follicle surrounding the crown may become thickened. Histologically, this thickened follicular fibrous tissue is often myxoid, with an abundant slightly basophilic ground substance, and commonly islands of odontogenic epithelium are also present (Fig. 57). Thus, the thickened follicle may have an appearance similar to that of odontogenic fibroma or myxoma, but if the tissue is from a relatively narrow zone surrounding the crown of an unerupted tooth it is likely to be a non-neoplastic thickened follicle rather than a fibroma or myxoma.

### 1.1.3.3 Benign Cementoblastoma (Cementoblastoma, True Cementoma)

*A neoplasm characterized by the formation of sheets of cementum-like tissue containing a large number of reversal lines and being unmineralized at the periphery of the mass or in the more active growth area.*

The benign cementoblastoma occurs almost always in the premolar or molar region, more commonly of the mandible than the maxilla, and there is a slight preponderance in males. Most cases are found in the 2nd and 3rd decades of life. Almost always, the tumour is closely related to and partly surrounds the root or roots of a single tooth.

Radiographically, the tumour is well defined and the central radiopacity is generally surrounded by a radiolucent zone of uniform width (Fig. 58) representing the peripheral unmineralized tissue and the formative cellular layers. Usually, the root of the associated tooth is shortened by resorption and the tumour hard tissue is fused to the root (Fig. 59). In the more mature parts of the growth the hard tissue contains a small number of entrapped cells, and the numerous strongly basophilic reversal lines (Fig. 60) give an appearance similar to that seen in Paget disease. The soft tissue component consists of vascular, loose-textured fibrous tissue containing large, deeply staining cells with a single nucleus and multinucleated cells. At the periphery (Fig. 61) and in other areas of active growth, extensive sheets of unmineralized tissue may be seen which show no remodelling. The newly formed unmineralized tissue at the periphery is often arranged in slender radiating columns (Fig. 61).

The lesion appears to be a benign neoplasm and is readily enucleated. Histologically, however, it may sometimes resemble an atypical osteosarcoma, and may also be difficult to distinguish from osteoid osteoma or osteoblastoma. However, it has the distinctive relationship to the root of a tooth and does not show the tendency to recur that has been found with osteoblastoma.

## 1.2 Malignant

### 1.2.1 Odontogenic Carcinomas

Most carcinomas found in the jaws have invaded from lesions of the oral mucosa. Some may be metastatic deposits from primary tumours in distant sites. Primary endosteal carcinoma of the jaws arises from epithelial residues in the jaws. As such epithelial remnants are of odontogenic origin, primary endosteal carcinomas of the jaws are referred to as odontogenic carcinomas.

Odontogenic carcinomas may develop by malignant transformation of an ameloblastoma or directly from residues of odontogenic epithelium following tooth development (so-called primary intraosseous carcinoma) or from the epithelial lining of odontogenic cysts. Subclassification of odontogenic carcinomas into these three categories is probably of academic and research interest only: from a clinicopathological point of view they are best considered together. Only by careful analysis of well-documented examples of each of the three categories would it be possible to determine whether there are any differences in their prognoses.

### 1.2.1.1 Malignant Ameloblastoma

*A neoplasm in which the pattern of an ameloblastoma and cytological features of malignancy are shown by the primary growth in the jaws and/or by any metastatic growth. Tumours meeting these criteria may arise as a result of malignant change in a pre-existing ameloblastoma, or possibly as a primary malignant ameloblastoma not preceded by an ordinary ameloblastoma.*

The histological features of a primary and a metastatic tumour are shown in Figs. 62–64.

The term 'malignant ameloblastoma' should not be applied to an ordinary ameloblastoma that endangers life through direct extension of the growth involving vital structures (e.g. extension into the base of the skull from a tumour of the maxilla).

Special care is needed in distinguishing between malignant ameloblastoma and intraosseous salivary gland tumours.

### 1.2.1.2 Primary Intraosseous Carcinoma

*A squamous cell carcinoma arising within the jaw, having no initial connection with the oral mucosa, and presumably developing from residues of the odontogenic epithelium.*

Some of the reported cases of primary intraosseous carcinoma of the jaws have shown histological features of squamous carcinoma which were indistinguishable from squamous carcinoma of the oral mucosa (Fig. 65). In such instances, a definitive diagnosis may be impossible without reliable clinical and radiological data. In other cases, however, the tumours have a distinctly odontogenic pattern (Fig. 66) with basal-type cells forming alveoli or arranged in a plexiform pattern with palisading of the peripheral cells. The nuclei of the latter are often orientated away from the basement membrane. There may be foci of squamous metaplasia or keratinization in these alveoli, similar to those seen in the acanthomatous variety of ameloblastoma.

Within the group of odontogenic carcinomas it is sometimes difficult to decide whether a tumour should be classified as a malignant ameloblastoma or as a primary intraosseous carcinoma. If there is histological evidence of a previous ameloblastoma at the site, the diagnosis of malignant ameloblastoma can be made with more confidence.

These lesions should not be difficult to distinguish from carcinomas arising from salivary tissue (particularly from intraosseous mucoepidermoid carcinoma).

#### 1.2.1.3 Malignant Variants of Other Odontogenic Epithelial Tumours

Whilst malignant ameloblastomas and primary intraosseous carcinomas are well documented, there is less evidence available concerning malignant variants of calcifying odontogenic cyst, calcifying epithelial odontogenic tumour and clear cell odontogenic tumour.

Tumours are known to occur which have features of calcifying odontogenic cyst, including varying numbers of ghost cells, and which also show cytological features and an infiltrative pattern suggestive of malignancy *(odontogenic ghost cell carcinoma).*

Calcifying epithelial odontogenic tumours commonly show cellular and nuclear pleomorphism, but these features do not necessarily indicate malignant behaviour with metastatic potential.

#### 1.2.1.4 Malignant Changes in Odontogenic Cysts

Although it has been suggested that keratinizing odontogenic cysts are more likely to become malignant than are non-keratinizing cysts, this has not been proven. It is clear, however, that malignant change in any form of odontogenic cyst is rare. Figures 67 and 68 illustrate epithelial dysplasia in a residual radicular cyst.

### 1.2.2 Odontogenic Sarcomas

#### 1.2.2.1 Ameloblastic Fibrosarcoma (Ameloblastic Sarcoma)

*A neoplasm with a similar structure to ameloblastic fibroma, but in which the ectomesenchymal component shows the features of a sarcoma.*

In the past, some of these rare tumours have been reported as 'malignant ameloblastomas'. However, the term 'ameloblastic fibrosarcoma' should be applied to those tumours in which it is the mesenchymal component, and not the odontogenic epithelium, that appears to be malignant (Figs. 69, 70).

#### 1.2.2.2 Ameloblastic Fibrodentinosarcoma and Ameloblastic Fibro-odontosarcoma

*Neoplasms similar to ameloblastic fibrosarcoma, but in which limited amounts of dysplastic dentine (dentinoid) have formed, and, in ameloblastic fibro-odontosarcoma, enamel as well.*

In the rare ameloblastic fibro-dentinosarcoma and fibro-odontosarcoma, parts of the odontogenic epithelium have exerted sufficient inductive influence to result in dentine formation, followed, in the odontosarcoma, by the deposition of enamel matrix, even though the ectomesenchymal component is sarcomatous. The presence of induced dentine and enamel does not appear to alter the basic nature of this neoplasm. Figure 71 shows the hard tissue formation and Figure 72 the sarcomatous mesenchymal component.

### 1.2.3 Odontogenic Carcinosarcoma

*A very rare neoplasm, similar in pattern to ameloblastic fibrosarcoma, but in which both the epithelial and the ectomesenchymal components show cytological features of malignancy.*

# 2 Neoplasms and Other Lesions Related to Bone

## 2.1 Osteogenic Neoplasms

### 2.1.1 Cemento-ossifying Fibroma (Cementifying Fibroma, Ossifying Fibroma)

*Demarcated or, rarely, encapsulated neoplasms consisting of fibrous tissue containing varying amounts of mineralized material resembling bone and/or cementum.*

These lesions may be difficult to distinguish from fibrous dysplasia, but they are sharply demarcated or rarely encapsulated masses that behave as benign neoplasms.

Radiographically, these neoplasms are well defined and contain varying amounts of radiopaque material (Fig. 73). The sharply defined character of the lesions is also apparent at operation (Fig. 74), and histologically the presence of this demarcation from the adjacent tissues is an important feature in distinguishing the tumours from fibrous dysplasia (Fig. 75). In the latter condition it is common to find that the metaplastic bone of the lesion is fused directly to the surrounding bone. In contrast, the hard tissues of cemento-ossifying fibromas do not fuse with the surrounding bone, except, occasionally, in limited areas.

Reference was made earlier to the difficulty of distinguishing between bone and cementum, and to the fact that both cementum and part of the bone of the jaws have a similar origin. Thus, the lesions in the cemento-ossifying fibroma group may be regarded as forming a continuous spectrum. The soft tissue component is a cellular fibrous tissue. Some of the lesions contain rounded or lobulated, strongly basophilic calcified masses (Fig. 76) with only occasional entrapped cells; these masses resemble atypical cementum. Other lesions contain trabeculae with the typical appearance of metaplastic bone, indistinguishable from that seen in fibrous dysplasia (Fig. 77). Some tumours in the group contain both cementum-like material and metaplastic bone in varying proportions. However, present evidence suggests that they all behave in a similar manner: unlike fibrous dysplasia, they continue to enlarge until removed.

The term *juvenile (aggressive) ossifying fibroma* is used for an actively growing lesion mainly affecting individuals below the age of 15 years. Juvenile ossifying fibroma consists of a cell-rich fibrous tissue containing bands of cellular osteoid without osteoblastic rimming together with trabeculae of more typical woven bone. Small foci of giant cells may be present, and in some parts there may be abundant osteoclasts related to the woven bone. Usually no fibrous capsule can be demonstrated, but like the ossifying fibroma described above (and unlike fibrous dysplasia), juvenile ossifying fibroma is well demarcated from the surrounding bone.

## 2.2 Non-neoplastic Bone Lesions

### 2.2.1 Fibrous Dysplasia of the Jaws

*A benign, self-limiting but non-encapsulated lesion occurring mainly in young subjects, usually in the maxilla, and showing replacement of the normal bone by a cellular fibrous tissue containing islands or trabeculae of metaplastic bone.*

Radiographically, the appearance depends upon the stage of the lesion. In the osteolytic stage there is an ill-defined radiolucency (Fig. 78), and in the later stages the progressive deposition of lesional bone results in a ground-glass appearance (Fig. 79). There is no sharp line of demarcation between lesional tissue and surrounding bone.

The histological pattern of the lesion varies with its age and stage of development. In the early lesion the tissue is fibroblastic, richly cellular (Fig. 80), and often shows a whorled pattern; there may be little bone. As the lesion progresses, the amount of bone increases (Fig. 81) and gradually the fibrous tissue decreases both in amount and in cellularity. The newly formed bone at the periphery fuses directly with the surrounding bone (Fig. 82), so that there is no capsule or line of demarcation except in limited areas. There may be cyst formation, and at some stages osteoclasts may be fairly numerous, but it is unusual to see substantial collections of multinucleated giant cells other than those directly related to the bone trabeculae. Some cementum-like tissue may be deposited, but cartilage is rarely, if ever, seen in fibrous dysplasia of the jaws.

Although fibrous dysplasia is self-limiting, the affected area does not return to normal. Radiographic change persists, and although the metaplastic bone of the active lesion will gradually be replaced by lamellar bone, this may have an abnormal and distinctive arrangement. The trabeculae of lamellar bone are slender, they tend to run parallel to one another, and they lie abnormally close together in a fibrous stroma that remains moderately cellular (Figs. 83, 84). The term *osseous keloid* has sometimes been used for lesions of this type.

Fibrous dysplasia of the jaws is usually a monostotic lesion, but may occasionally be part of a polyostotic process.

### 2.2.2 Cemento-osseous Dysplasias

There is a variety of jaw lesions that are characterized histologically by the presence of cementum-like tissue, and which (unlike cemento-ossifying fibroma) appear to be dysplasias rather than neoplasms. These cemento-osseous dysplasias present both clinically and histopathologically in a number of forms, and the relationship between them is uncertain; some authorities regard them as forming part of a continuous spectrum, and others regard them as separate entities. Whilst recognizing these differing points of view, in the context of the present publication it is useful to describe certain more or less well-defined clinicopathological presentations, without rejecting the possibility that they may be related to one another.

#### 2.2.2.1 Periapical Cemental Dysplasia (Periapical Fibrous Dysplasia)

*A non-neoplastic lesion affecting the periapical tissues of one or more teeth, and with histological features similar to those of the lesions of the cemento-ossifying fibroma group, but without a sharply defined margin.*

This lesion is most easily recognized when it affects the periapical areas of several teeth (Fig. 85), which may be adjacent to one another or in different parts of the jaws. A common presentation is in the mandibular incisor region in middle-aged women. Mainly fibroblastic in the early stages, there is progressive deposition of metaplastic bone, cementum-like tissue or both (Fig. 86). Each periapical lesion is self-limiting, rarely exceeds 1 cm in diameter, and ultimately becomes a dense mineralized mass (Fig. 85).

#### 2.2.2.2 Florid Cemento-osseous Dysplasia (Gigantiform Cementoma, Familial Multiple Cementomas)

*Lobulated masses of dense, highly mineralized, almost acellular cemento-osseous tissue typically occurring in several parts of the jaws. Black persons are affected more commonly than white, and sometimes there is a familial distribution.*

These radiographically dense masses (Fig. 87) are sometimes distributed more or less symmetrically in the jaws, which supports the view that they represent some form of dysplasia or developmental anomaly. However, the masses may attain a considerable size and cause expansion of the jaw. Histologically, the lesion consists of large sheets or fused globules of cemento-osseous tissue (Fig. 88), sometimes strongly basophilic, which may be fused to the roots of one or more teeth or may lie separately. When fused to the roots, florid cemento-osseous dysplasia must be distinguished from hypercementosis, in which abnormal amounts of cellular cementum are laid down in an orderly manner on the root of the tooth. It should be noted that masses similar to those of florid cemento-osseous dysplasia may form in the jaws in some cases of Paget disease.

#### 2.2.2.3 Other Cemento-osseous Dysplasias

*Lesions which share some of the features of periapical cemental dysplasia and/or florid cemento-osseous dysplasia, but do not have their characteristic clinicopathological patterns of presentation.*

### 2.2.3 Cherubism (Familial Multilocular Cystic Disease of the Jaws)

*A benign, self-limiting condition in which the lesional tissue consists of vascular fibrous tissue containing varying numbers of multinucleated giant cells arranged diffusely or focally.*

The lesions occur in children, sometimes early in childhood, and usually show a familial tendency. They affect one or more quadrants of the jaws, forming radiolucent, usually multilocular, areas and expanding the bone (Figs. 89, 90).

The bone lesions are more active in younger patients; after the age of about 12 years activity usually diminishes and finally the lesions become inactive. Consequently the histological findings vary. The more active lesion is cellular with many giant cells (Fig. 91) and may contain multiple foci of extravasated blood. In some cases a cuff of acidophilic van Gieson-positive material is seen around the vessels (Fig. 92). As activity diminishes the lesional tissue becomes progressively more fibrous, the number of giant cells diminishes, and new bone is laid down.

### 2.2.4 Central Giant Cell Granuloma

*An intraosseous lesion consisting of more or less cellular fibrous tissue containing multiple foci of haemorrhage, aggregations of multinucleated giant cells, and sometimes trabeculae of woven bone forming within the septa of more mature fibrous tissue that may traverse the lesion.*

Giant cell granuloma may occur in either jaw and at any age. It is seen most commonly, however, in the tooth-bearing area of the mandible in the 3rd decade of life.

Radiographically, there is an area of bone destruction which has a smooth or lobulated outline (Fig. 93 a) and which may be traversed by slender bony septa resulting in a multilocular pattern (Fig. 93 b). The radiographic appearance may thus bear some similarity to that of an ameloblastoma. The histological pattern varies considerably. In some cases, the focal aggregation of giant cells is clear (Figs. 94,

95) and trabeculae of bone often extend between the foci of giant cells (Fig. 96). In others, the tissue is loose-textured and oedematous and the giant cells may show little evidence of a focal arrangement. Fresh haemorrhage is a frequent feature and deposits of fibrinoid material may also be seen. Haemosiderin may be scanty or abundant, and mitoses are not uncommon.

The lesion can expand the bone and penetrate the cortex, sometimes presenting as a gingival swelling. In these instances the superficial aspect appears encapsulated, but on the deeper aspect the relationship with the bone is irregular. Removal is sometimes followed by recurrence, but the lesion is not invasive and does not metastasize. In some very cell-rich areas the lesion may resemble a giant cell tumour, whilst other examples contain a few relatively large blood spaces, though not so large as those commonly found in the aneurysmal bone cyst.

It may be impossible to distinguish on histological grounds between the giant cell granuloma, cherubism, and the brown node of hyperparathyroidism.

Distinction between true giant cell tumour and giant cell granuloma may be difficult. Comparison of the giant cells in giant cell granuloma of the jaws and in giant cell tumours of long bones has shown that the giant cells in giant cell granulomas tend to be smaller and to contain fewer nuclei. Well-documented true giant cell tumours do occur in the jaws: like the long bone lesions they contain larger giant cells with greater numbers of nuclei.

### 2.2.5 Aneurysmal Bone Cyst

*A benign intraosseous lesion, characterized by blood-filled spaces of varying size associated with a fibroblastic tissue containing multinucleated giant cells, osteoid, and woven bone.*

Aneurysmal bone cyst of the jaws usually occurs in individuals below the age of 30 years, more often in the mandible than in the maxilla. There is a slight female preponderance.

Radiographically, it is a radiolucent lesion, sometimes of a multiloculated appearance, which balloons the cortex (Fig. 97).

Histologically, there are many large and small cavernous spaces filled with erythrocytes (Fig. 98). The spaces are usually contained within a cellular connective tissue with fresh and old haemorrhages, which may show organization, numerous multinucleated giant cells, haemosiderin, and slender trabeculae of osteoid (Figs. 99, 100). The solid areas with large numbers of giant cells and fibroblasts, together with foci of haemorrhage and of haemosiderin deposition, may look very much like giant cell granuloma of the jaws. Other solid areas may have the appearance of fibrous dysplasia, cemento-ossifying fibroma, and possibly other jaw tumours. These so-called 'hybrid lesions' give support to the view that aneurysmal bone cyst may represent secondary change in a pre-existing lesion.

### 2.2.6 Solitary Bone Cyst (Traumatic, Simple, Haemorrhagic Bone Cyst)

*An intraosseous cyst having a tenuous lining of connective tissue with no epithelium.*

The solitary bone cyst is most often seen during the second decade of life, and cases are rarely seen after the age of 25 years. The most common locations in the jaws are the body and symphyseal area of the mandible.

Radiographically, the solitary bone cyst presents as a well-defined unilocular radiolucent area (Fig. 101), often with a scalloping of the margin between the roots of the premolars and molars or in areas remote from the teeth.

Histologically, the solitary bone cyst has no epithelial lining. The bony walls are covered by a thin, loose-textured fibrous tissue (Fig. 102) that may contain multinucleated giant cells and haemosiderin granules. Although sometimes termed a 'traumatic' or 'haemorrhagic' bone cyst, the pathogenesis of this lesion is unknown.

## 2.3 Other Tumours

### 2.3.1 Melanotic Neuroectodermal Tumour of Infancy (Melanotic Progonoma)

*A tumour arising, typically, in the anterior part of the maxilla in an infant under the age of 1 year. The tumour consists of varying proportions of two cell types – epithelium-like cells, often arranged in strands, and small, darkly staining lymphocyte-like cells – in a cellular, fibrous stroma. Melanin is found within the epithelium-like cells, and to a lesser extent within the lymphocyte-like cells.*

On the basis of embryological, ultrastructural and biochemical evidence it is now assumed that this tumour is derived from cells of neural crest origin.

The lesion may be present as a pigmented or non-pigmented exophytic gingival tumour or it may be contained within the bone. The area of bone destruction may be traversed by bone septa, and the associated developing teeth are often displaced (Fig. 103). The cut surface of the lesional tissue shows pigmentation varying from mottled grey patches to a uniform deep black. The epithelium-like cells and the lymphocyte-like cells may appear in separate areas of the lesion, though more commonly they are together (Fig. 104). The epithelium-like cells are often pale-staining; they may be arranged in sheets, cords, or duct-like structures, and the latter may contain lymphocyte-like cells within the ducts or clefts (Fig. 105). Melanin granules may be scanty or the cells may be heavily loaded (Fig. 106).

The appearance of the lymphocyte-like cells varies considerably. In some instances they resemble small lymphocytes, with a dense, rounded nucleus and little cytoplasm (Fig. 104). In other instances the nucleus is larger, with a finer chromatin pattern. At the margins the tumour sometimes extends irregularly into the bone, so that the lesion appears invasive, but recurrence is very rare. Only a few malignant examples have been reported.

A small number of cases of an apparently identical tumour have been reported in the mandible and in several other parts of the body.

# 3 Epithelial Cysts

## 3.1 Developmental

### 3.1.1 Odontogenic

#### 3.1.1.1 "Gingival Cysts" of Infants (Epstein Pearls)

*Small cysts arising from epithelial cell rests in the alveolar mucosa of infants.*

These lesions, which are commonly present at birth, are seldom seen over the age of 3 months. They are white or yellow nodules and are found over the future tooth-bearing area of the alveolar mucosa.

Histologically there is a thin lining of stratified squamous epithelium with flat basal cells and a parakeratinized surface. Keratin fills the cyst cavity (Fig. 107).

### 3.1.1.2 Odontogenic Keratocyst (Primordial Cyst)

*A cyst arising in the tooth-bearing areas of the jaws, or posterior to the mandibular third molar, and characterized by a thin fibrous capsule and a lining of keratinized stratified squamous epithelium usually about five to eight cells in thickness and generally without rete ridges.*

This type of cyst is thought to arise from the dental lamina or its remnants, or from offshoots of the basal layer of oral epithelium. The stimulus to cyst formation is unknown, but it is not inflammation.

The lesions occur over a wide age range with a peak frequency in the 2nd and 3rd decades and a second peak in the 5th decade. They are more common in male than in female subjects.

The mandible is involved much more frequently than the maxilla. About half of the cases occur at the angle of the mandible and extend for varying distances into the ramus and forward into the body. There is no special relationship to a tooth.

Radiographically, the keratocyst may show a unilocular or multilocular pattern and the cystic spaces may have a smooth or scalloped border (Fig. 108).

Histologically, the cyst wall is thin unless there is inflammation. The basal layer of the epithelium is well defined and is composed of either columnar or cuboidal cells (Fig. 109). The keratinization of the epithelium is predominantly of the parakeratotic type, but cases with orthokeratosis are seen. Often the cyst lining has a corrugated surface (Fig. 110), and in some specimens the epithelial lining in part of the wall becomes detached from the fibrous capsule (Fig. 111). Occasionally the epithelium shows features of dysplasia. In some odontogenic keratocysts the connective tissue contains islands of epithelium or separate daughter cysts (Fig. 112). If inflammation supervenes the fibrous capsule becomes thickened, the epithelium develops rete processes, and the keratinization may be lost (Fig. 113).

The pathologist may also receive material aspirated from a suspected keratocyst. Smears prepared from this material are likely to show squames; because these are not freshly shed but have been trapped within the cyst for a considerable time, they often show partial breakdown and ill-defined margins (Fig. 114).

A keratocyst may envelop an adjacent unerupted tooth (envelopmental keratocyst; Fig. 108 a). Sometimes a tooth may erupt into the cavity of a keratocyst (follicular keratocyst). Such cases may be erroneously diagnosed as dentigerous cyst with a keratinizing lining.

Most keratocysts are isolated lesions, but similar cysts also occur as part of the multiple naevoid basal cell carcinoma and jaw cyst syndrome. In this condition the keratocysts are commonly multiple (Fig. 115).

Odontogenic keratocysts have a marked tendency to recur.

#### 3.1.1.3 Dentigerous (Follicular) Cyst

*A cyst which encloses the crown and is attached to the neck of an unerupted tooth. It develops by accumulation of fluid between the reduced enamel epithelium and the crown, or between the layers of the reduced enamel epithelium.*

Dentigerous cysts are most often found in relation to the mandibular third molar, the maxillary canine and third molar, and the mandibular second premolar. They occur at all ages but most frequently in the 2nd, 3rd and 4th decades, and more frequently in male than in female subjects.

Radiographically, a dentigerous cyst is seen as a well-defined radiolucent area associated with the crown of an unerupted tooth (Fig. 116). Often the radiolucent area surrounds the crown, but sometimes it lies mainly or entirely to one side. In Fig. 117 the cyst associated with a maxillary canine has been opened to show the attachment at the neck of the tooth.

Histologically, the cyst wall is composed of a thin layer of connective tissue lined by epithelium that may be only two to three cells thick (Fig. 118 a) and this resembles the reduced enamel epithelium. If there is inflammation the epithelium becomes thicker and more squamous. The lining epithelium may include a variable number of mucus-producing cells (Fig. 118 b) and sometimes also ciliated cells. In some cases the cyst lining is keratinized, although generally such keratinization is only in limited areas. In the adjacent connective tissue, islands of odontogenic epithelium are often seen, and these appear inactive.

#### 3.1.1.4 Eruption Cyst

*A cyst that surrounds the crown of an erupting tooth, lies partly outside the bone, and is lined by non-keratinizing stratified squamous epithelium.*

The eruption cyst is a form of dentigerous cyst lying in soft tissues external to the bone. Clinically it presents as a bluish swelling in an area where a tooth will erupt.

The histological appearance is shown in Fig. 119. The chronic inflammatory infiltrate adjacent to the epithelium is a result of occlusal trauma and leads to proliferation and thickening of the epithelial lining.

#### 3.1.1.5 Lateral Periodontal Cyst

*A cyst occurring on the lateral aspect or between the roots of vital teeth and arising from odontogenic epithelial remnants, but not as a result of inflammatory stimuli.*

The lateral periodontal cyst must be distinguished from a collateral odontogenic keratocyst, from a gingival cyst of adults and from a cyst of inflammatory origin lateral to the root of the tooth.

The most frequent location is the premolar area of the mandible, followed by the anterior region of the maxilla. There is a wide age distribution. Radiographs show a well-defined round or ovoid radiolucent area, occasionally with a sclerotic margin (Fig. 120).

Lateral periodontal cysts arise from odontogenic epithelium, but precisely from which part is controversial. Reduced enamel epithelium, remnants of dental lamina and cell rests of Malassez have been implicated.

The cysts are lined by a thin, non-keratinizing squamous or cuboidal epithelium, ranging from one to five cell layers thick (Fig. 121). Nuclei are small and pyknotic. Localized epithelial plaques or thickenings, which may be rounded or flattened, and consisting of fusiform or water-clear cells, are frequently seen (Figs. 121, 122).

The so-called *botryoid odontogenic cyst* is probably a multilocular variant of the lateral periodontal cyst (Fig. 123).

#### 3.1.1.6 Gingival Cyst of Adults

*A cyst arising from odontogenic epithelial remnants and involving the gingiva of adults.*

The cysts are well-circumscribed swellings, usually less than 1 cm in diameter, which occur in the attached gingiva or interdental papilla and almost always on the facial aspect. They are most commonly seen in the canine-premolar region of the mandible. There may be no radiographic change or only a faint round shadow indicative of superficial bone erosion.

Their origin is controversial, but remnants of dental lamina and junctional epithelium from adjacent teeth have been implicated. The lining of the cyst varies from an extremely thin epithelium with one or two layers of flat or cuboidal cells, to a rather thicker stratified squamous epithelium without rete ridges (Figs. 124, 125). In some cysts, localized epithelial plaques of fusiform or water-clear cells have been described, similar to those found in the lateral periodontal cyst.

### 3.1.1.7 Glandular Odontogenic Cyst; Sialo-odontogenic Cyst

*A cyst arising in the tooth-bearing areas of the jaws and characterized by an epithelial lining with cuboidal or columnar cells both at the surface and lining crypts or cyst-like spaces within the thickness of the epithelium.*

This type of cyst has been characterized only recently, and few examples have been reported. As yet there is no general agreement on the most suitable name for the lesion; two suggestions are given above. The lesion arises within the bone of either jaw. It grows slowly but may reach a considerable size, and with the larger examples there appears to be a tendency to recurrence.

The fibrous capsule is usually free from inflammatory cells. The lining epithelium may be partly squamous and without distinctive features. However, in more or less extensive areas the stratified epithelium has a surface layer of acidophilic cuboidal or columnar cells, often forming irregular papillary projections. These surface cells include a variable number that are ciliated, and similarly variable numbers are mucus-producing. Within the thickness of the epithelium there may be crypts or cyst-like spaces lined by cells like those seen at the epithelial surface (Figs. 126, 127). Mucin may be demonstrable within the intraepithelial spaces and within the main cyst cavity. Epithelial plaques may be present, similar to those seen in the lateral periodontal cyst and the gingival cyst of adults. Multilocular or botryoid varieties also occur.

It should be emphasized that many types of odontogenic cyst show areas of mucous cell or ciliated cell metaplasia; in the absence of the pattern described above, the presence of such areas should not lead to the diagnosis of glandular odontogenic cyst.

## 3.1.2 Non-odontogenic

### 3.1.2.1 Nasopalatine Duct (Incisive Canal) Cyst

*A cyst arising from the epithelial residues in the nasopalatine (incisive) canal.*

Most cases occur in the 4th, 5th and 6th decades, and there is a three-to-one preponderance in males as compared to females.

Radiographically, the cyst is found in the midline of the maxilla as a well-defined round, ovoid or heart-shaped radiolucency (Fig. 128). On occlusal radiographs the cyst appears behind the incisors.

Histologically, the cyst may be lined by stratified squamous epithelium, pseudostratified ciliated columnar epithelium (Fig. 129), or both. Transitional types of epithelium may also be found, depending upon the presence of inflammation in the adjacent connective tissue. The connective tissue in the wall of nasopalatine duct cysts characteristically contains large nerves and vessels; mucous glands and adipose tissue may also be present (Fig. 130), and a small island of hyaline cartilage is sometimes included.

An extraosseous presentation of this lesion, which arises in the same epithelial residues but superficial to the nasopalatine canal, is termed *cyst of the palatine papilla.*

### 3.1.2.2 Nasolabial (Nasoalveolar) Cyst

*A cyst situated on the alveolar process near the base of the nostril.*

There is a wide age distribution of this lesion, with a peak frequency in the 4th and 5th decades. There is a considerable preponderance in females.

The cyst does not arise within the bone, but may cause superficial erosion of the outer surface of the maxilla. Radiographically, it may not be recognized unless demonstrated by injection of radiopaque material.

The most likely origin of the nasolabial cyst is thought to be remnants of the embryonic nasolacrimal duct or the lower anterior portion of the mature duct.

The wall of the enucleated cyst is commonly corrugated (Fig. 131). The cyst is most frequently lined by non-ciliated pseudostratified columnar epithelium (Fig. 132), which may contain abundant mucous cells (Fig. 131). There may be localized areas of squamous epithelium or cuboidal epithelium.

## Note

Various non-odontogenic cysts of the mouth and jaws were thought to arise from epithelium trapped in the lines of fusion of the embryonic processes. Now, however, it is generally believed that the grooves between the processes are not eliminated by side-to-side fusion, and that epithelium is unlikely to become trapped. Critical re-examination of the so-called 'fissural' cysts suggests that many of the types previously recognized do not exist as separate entities. These debatable lesions are listed and commented on below, but they are not included in the formal classification.

**Median Palatine, Median Alveolar and Median Mandibular Cysts**

*Midline cysts of the maxilla and mandible, previously thought to be entities derived from epithelium entrapped during the fusion of embryonic facial processes.*

The existence of these cysts as entities derived in this way has been seriously questioned by embryologists and pathologists. It is now felt that those in the maxilla represent a posterior extension of a nasopalatine duct cyst in the case of a median palatine cyst and an anterior extension in the case of a median alveolar cyst. Occasionally, a cyst in the median alveolar position is a keratocyst. Cysts in the midline of the mandible may be radicular cysts, lateral periodontal cysts or odontogenic keratocysts.

**Globulomaxillary Cyst**

*A cyst found within the bone between the maxillary lateral incisor and canine, previously thought to be a fissural cyst arising from non-odontogenic epithelium included at the site of fusion of the globular process of the frontonasal process and the maxillary process.*

Radiographically, a cyst in the globulomaxillary area shows a characteristic inverted pear-shaped radiolucency between the lateral incisor and canine, occasionally causing divergence of the roots.

The concept of a globulomaxillary cyst formed by the entrapment of epithelium during development of the face has been seriously questioned. Cysts undoubtedly occur in this region, and the majority probably represent a range of other varieties, such as the odontogenic keratocyst, lateral radicular or residual cysts, and lateral periodontal cysts. However, a few cysts in this particular location are not readily placed in any of these other categories.

# 3.2 Inflammatory

## 3.2.1 Radicular Cyst

*A cyst arising from the epithelial residues (rests of Malassez) in the periodontal ligament as a consequence of inflammation, usually following the death of the dental pulp.*

#### 3.2.1.1 Apical and Lateral Radicular Cyst

These radicular cysts are the most common cysts found in the jaws. They develop when a pulpal inflammation spreads to the periapical or lateral radicular area and gives rise to the formation of an apical or lateral granuloma. Within a granuloma, epithelial residues (rests of Malassez), stimulated by the inflammation, may proliferate and lead to the formation of an epithelium-lined cystic cavity.

The radicular cyst may occur in relation to any tooth, but few are associated with the deciduous dentition. The highest incidence is in the anterior region of the maxilla. They are found over a wide age range, with a peak in the 3rd and 4th decades. Male subjects are affected more frequently than female.

Radiographically, it is not always possible to differentiate between a radicular cyst and an apical granuloma, although cysts tend to be larger and to have well-defined margins (Fig. 133).

Histologically, most radicular cysts are lined by non-keratinized stratified squamous epithelium (Fig. 134). The morphology of the epithelium is dependent upon the degree of inflammation. In the presence of inflammation, the cyst epithelium will show proliferating rete processes (Fig. 135). When inflammation is absent, the epithelium tends to be thin with no rete processes, and there may be more or less extensive juxtaepithelial hyalinization (Fig. 136). When the hyalinization is extensive, the epithelium becomes tenuous and degenerate (Fig. 137). Occasionally the cyst epithelium contains mucous or ciliated cells, even in mandibular radicular cysts. Hyaline bodies of characteristic appearance are seen in some cases (Figs. 138, 139) and may become calcified.

Foam cells may be seen in the cystic cavity (Fig. 140). In the fibrous cyst wall there are often heavy deposits of cholesterol crystals with an associated foreign-body giant cell reaction. The inflammatory cell infiltrate is mixed and may include foam cells and plasma cells with prominent Russell bodies. Commonly, the wall of the radicular cyst has a zone heavily infiltrated with inflammatory cells, between the epithelial lining and an outer fibrous zone with fewer inflammatory cells.

#### 3.2.1.2 Residual Radicular Cyst

*A radicular cyst which is retained in the jaws after removal of the associated tooth (Fig. 141).*

### 3.2.2 Paradental (Inflammatory Collateral, Mandibular Infected Buccal) Cyst

*A cyst occurring near to the cervical margin of the lateral aspect of a root as a consequence of an inflammatory process in a periodontal pocket (Fig. 142).*

The paradental cyst arises from odontogenic epithelium in the superficial part of the periodontal ligament; the involved tooth is vital.

A distinctive form of the paradental cyst occurs on the buccal and distal aspects of erupted mandibular molars, most commonly the third molars, where there is an associated history of pericoronitis.

Similar cysts, almost all of which occur on the buccal surface of the mandibular first molars in children around 6–8 years of age, have been described as the *mandibular infected buccal cyst.*

The histological features of the inflammatory paradental cyst are the same as those of the radicular cyst.

#### Note

As previously indicated, the lining of many cysts of the jaws, both odontogenic and developmental, may include ciliated epithelium. However, when a specimen from a suspected cyst of the maxilla is mainly lined by ciliated epithelium, consideration should be given to the possibility that the material is antral lining, or the lining of a *postoperative maxillary cyst (surgical ciliated cyst)* formed at the site of a previous operation involving the antrum.

# Subject Index

Unless otherwise stated, all the preparations shown in the photomicrographs on the following pages were stained with haematoxylin and eosin.

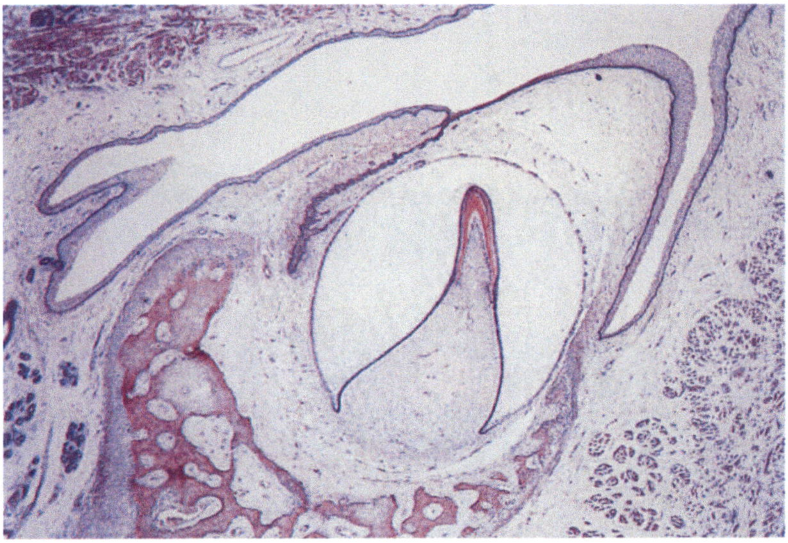

**Fig. 1.** Tooth germ in a fetus of about 4.5 months of age. Developing deciduous lower central incisor. ×20

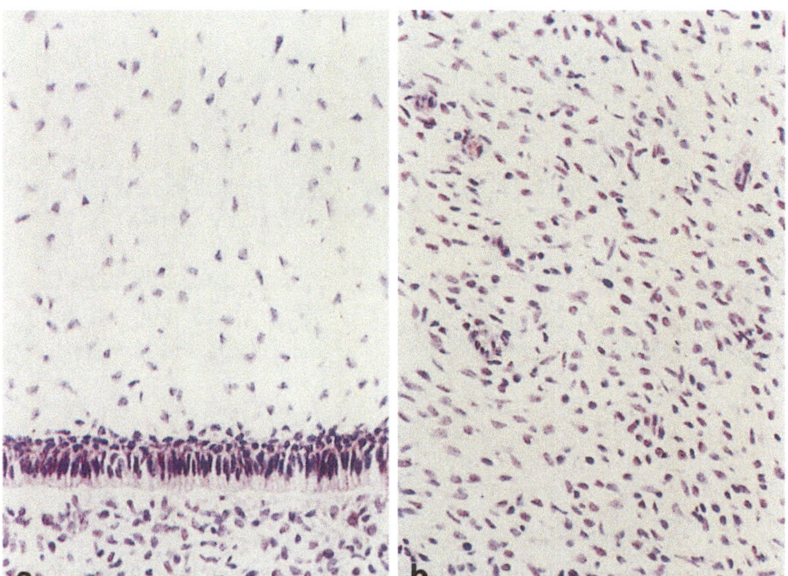

**Fig. 2.** **a** Stellate reticulum of enamel organ. Stellate reticulum with stratum intermedium and ameloblast layer below. ×320. **b** Dental papilla. ×320

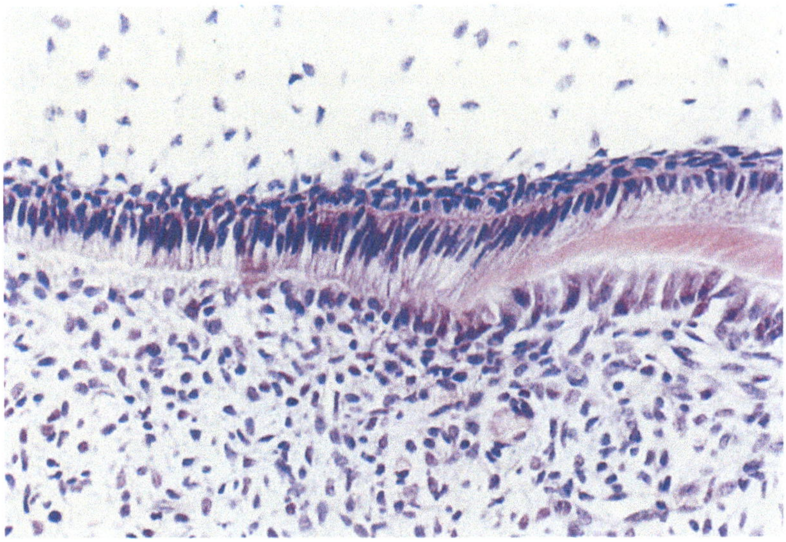

**Fig. 3.** Enamel organ *(above)* and dental papilla *(below)*. Odontoblasts have differentiated and some dentine has formed. ×320

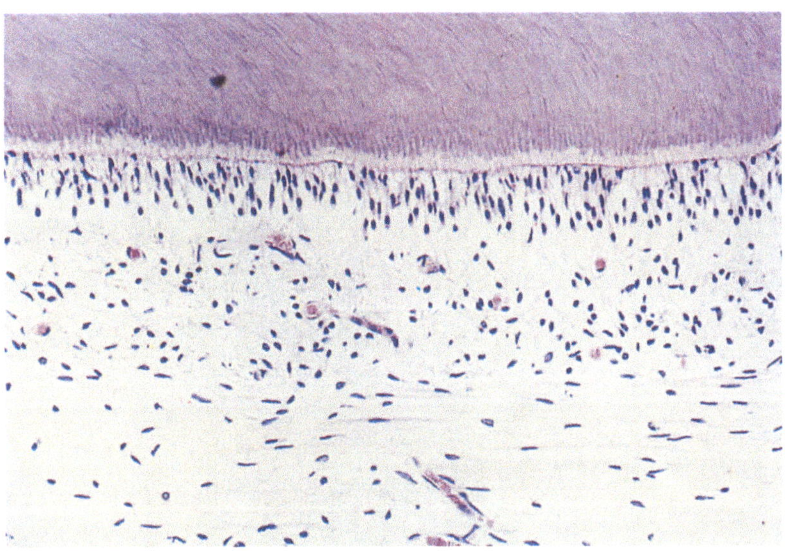

**Fig. 4.** Dentine and pulp in fully formed tooth. The pseudostratified odontoblast layer lies at the surface of the pulp. ×200

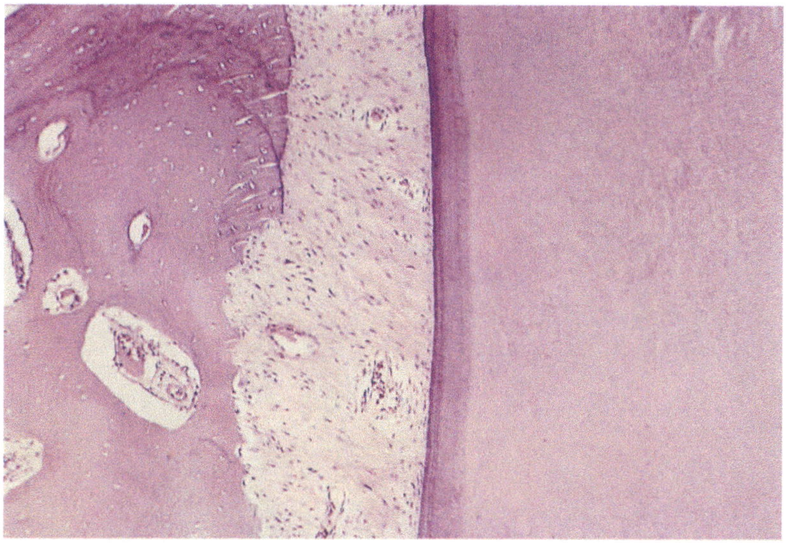

**Fig. 5.** Acellular cementum. From *left* to *right:* bone, periodontal ligament, cementum and dentine. ×80

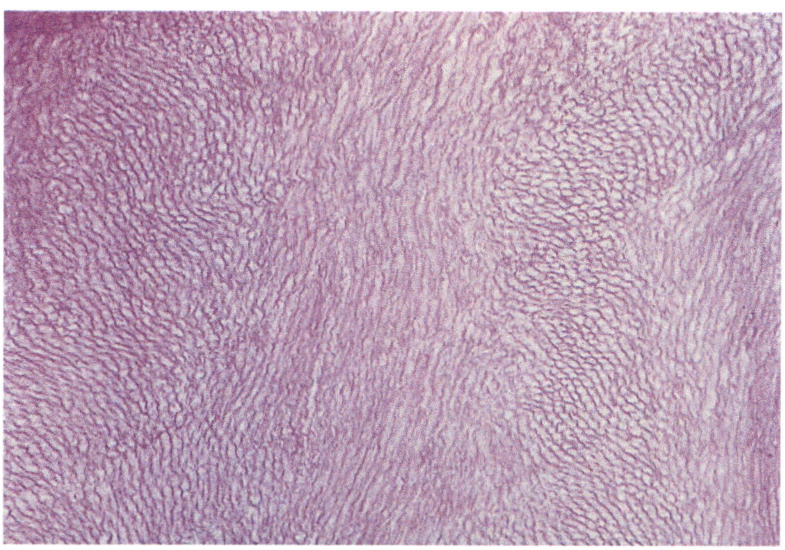

**Fig. 6.** Enamel matrix. Tenuous matrix remaining after demineralization shows outlines of enamel prisms cut in varying directions. ×320

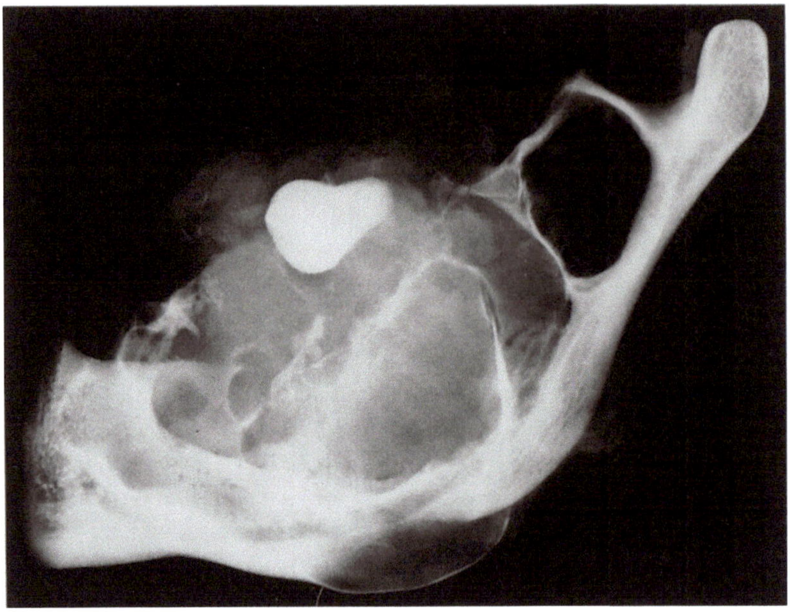

**Fig. 7.** *Ameloblastoma,* mandible. Resection specimen showing multilocular radiolucency and displacement of a molar tooth

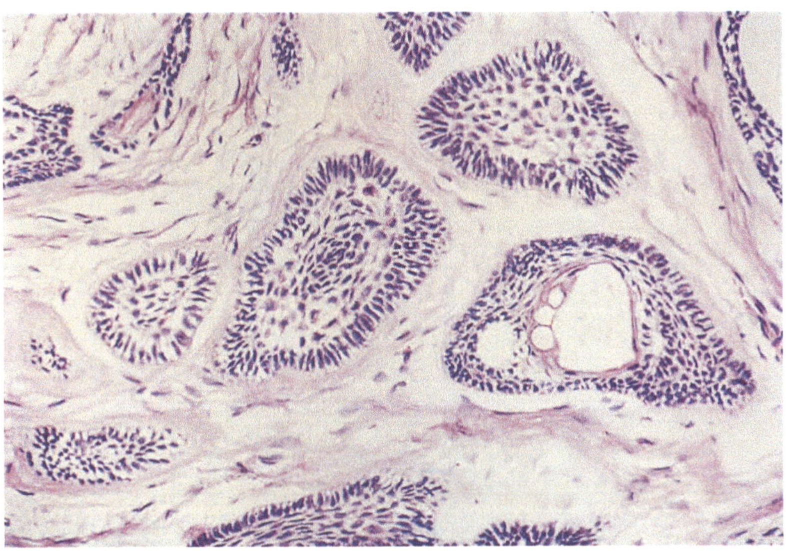

**Fig. 8.** *Ameloblastoma, follicular.* Epithelial islands bounded by columnar cells. ×200

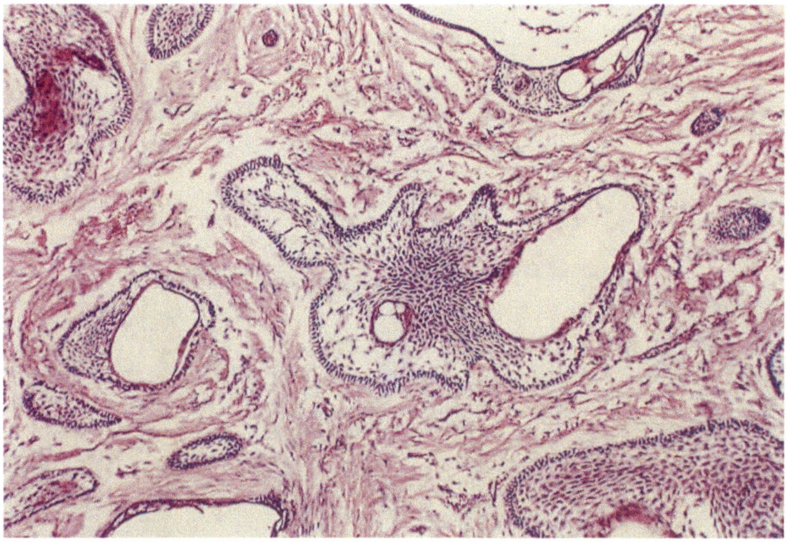

**Fig. 9.** *Ameloblastoma, follicular.* Many epithelial islands show early cyst formation. × 80

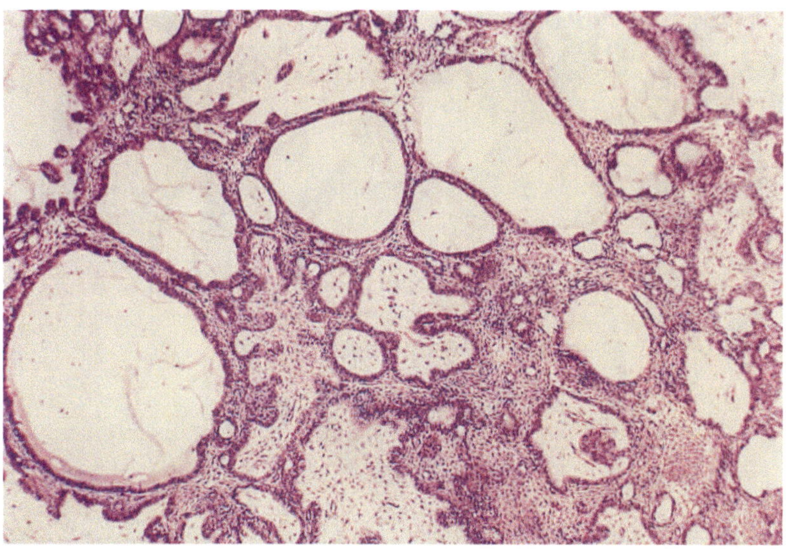

**Fig. 10.** *Ameloblastoma, plexiform.* Continuous meshwork of epithelium and cysts resulting from stromal degeneration. × 80

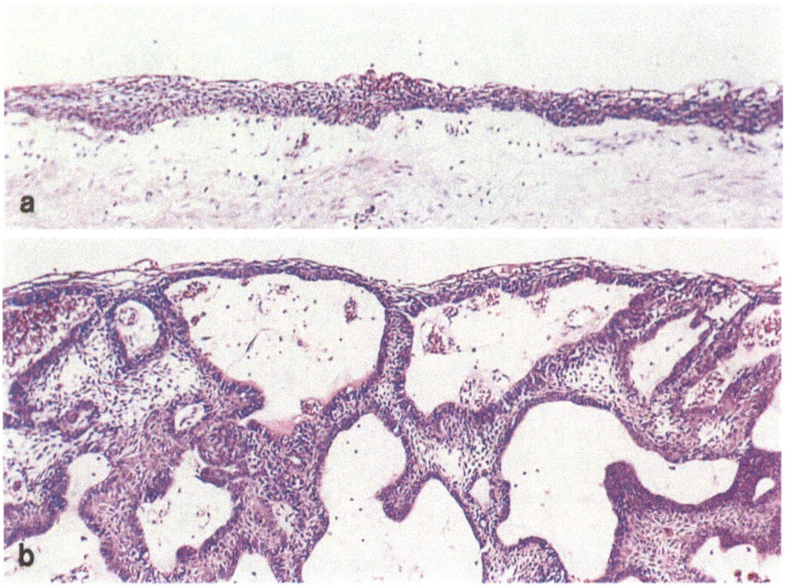


**Fig. 11 a, b.** *Unicystic ameloblastoma.* **a** Thin cyst lining. × 80. **b** Another part of the same cyst, showing typical plexiform ameloblastoma pattern. × 80

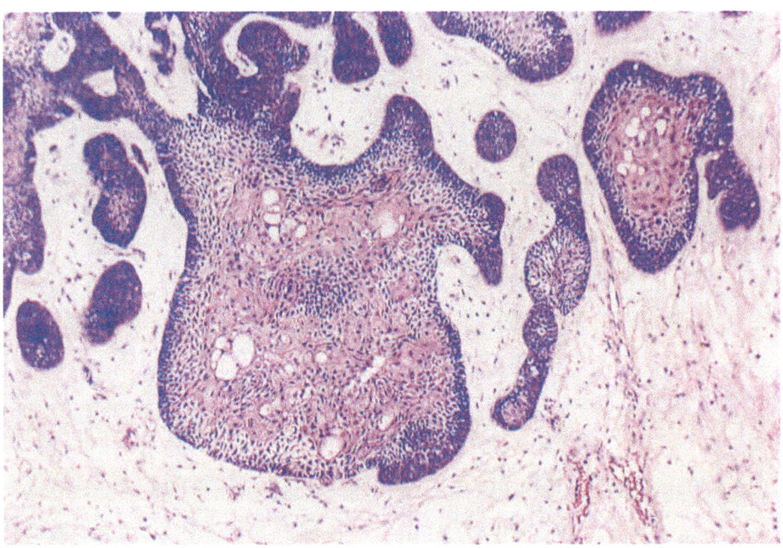

**Fig. 12.** *Ameloblastoma, follicular.* Acanthomatous type showing squamous metaplasia. × 80

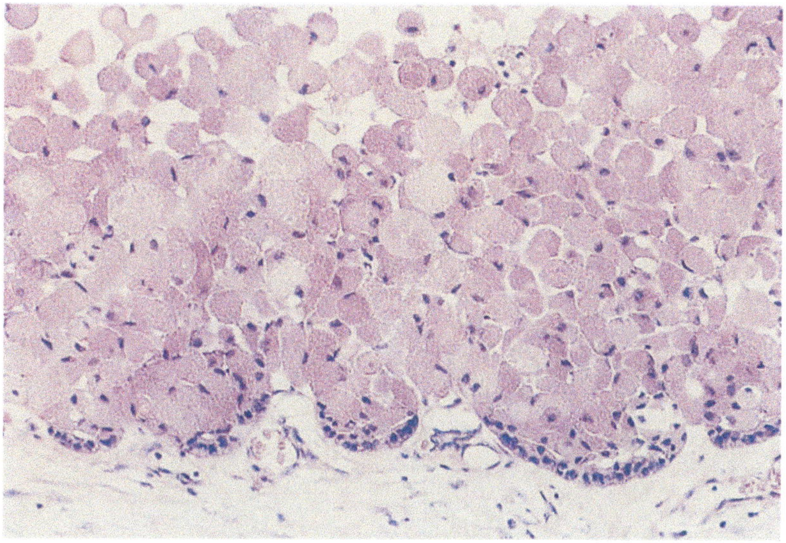

**Fig. 13.** *Ameloblastoma, granular cell type.* Rounded cells packed with acidophilic granules. Columnar cells are still present at the margin. ×200

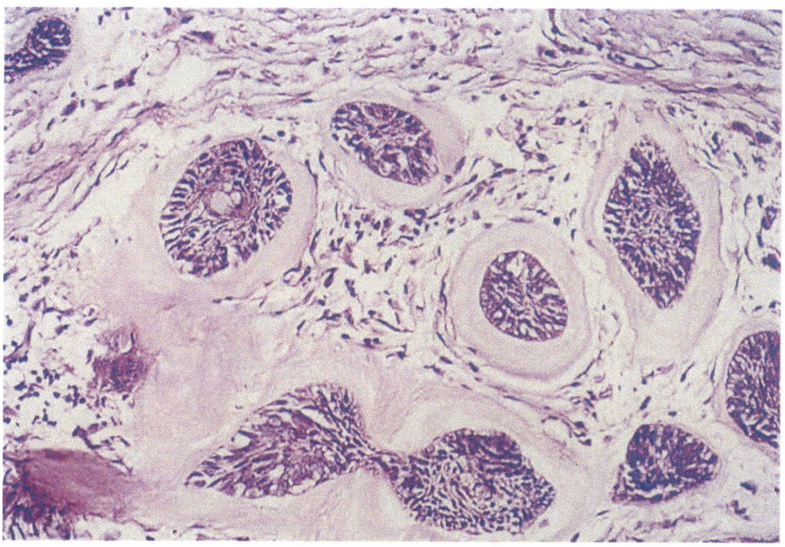

**Fig. 14.** *Ameloblastoma, follicular.* Marked juxtaepithelial hyalinization. ×200

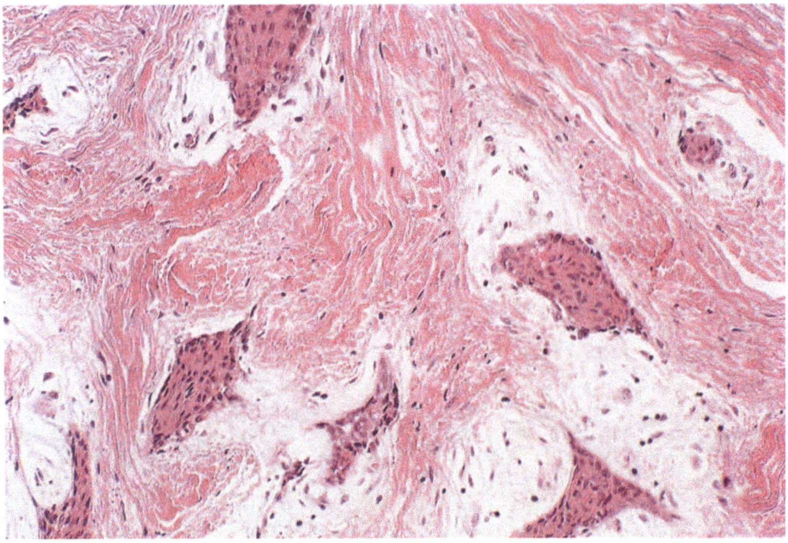

**Fig. 15.** *Ameloblastoma, desmoplastic.* ×160

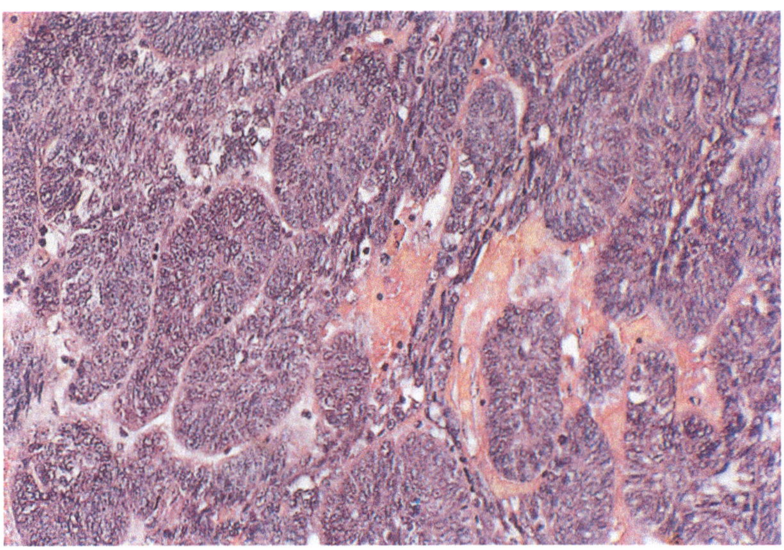

**Fig. 16.** *Ameloblastoma, basaloid pattern.* ×200

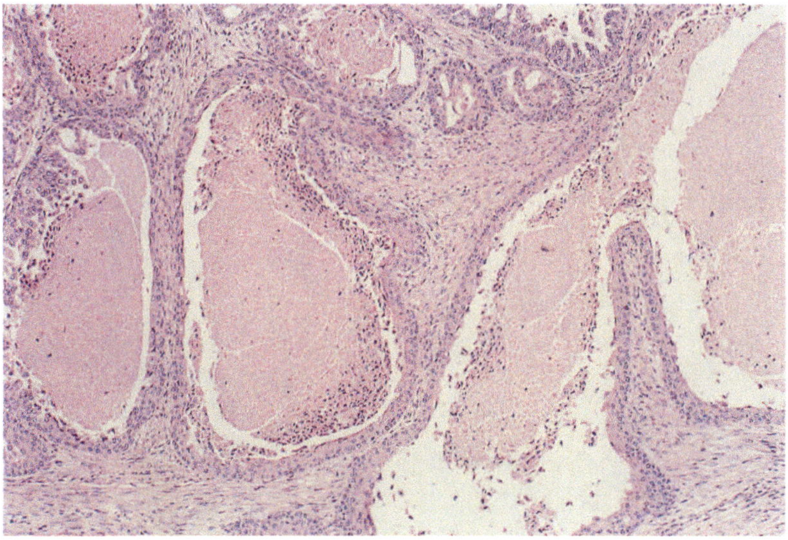

**Fig. 17.** *Papilliferous keratoameloblastoma.* × 80

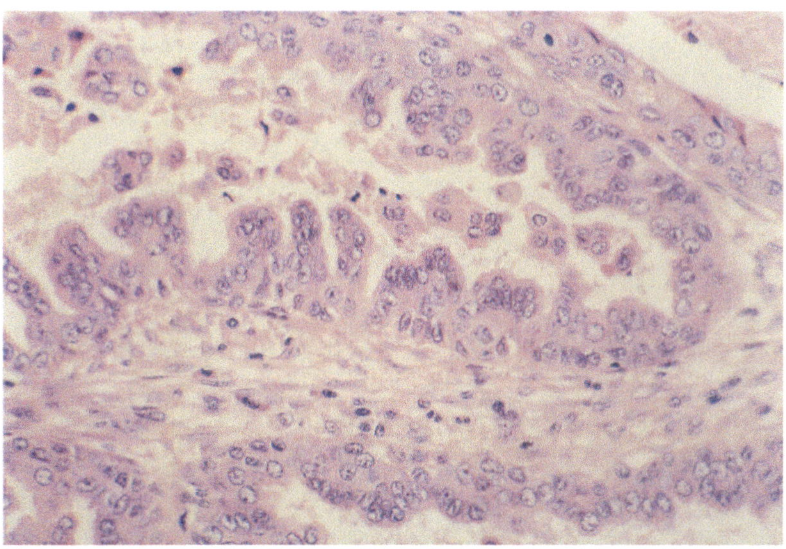

**Fig. 18.** *Papilliferous keratoameloblastoma.* × 320

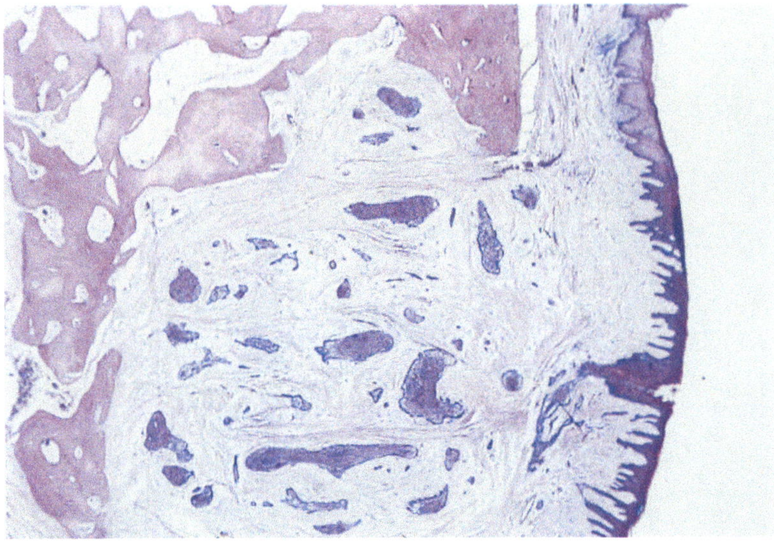

**Fig. 19.** *Ameloblastoma, peripheral.* Small tumour beneath mucosa, causing resorption of underlying bone. ×12.5

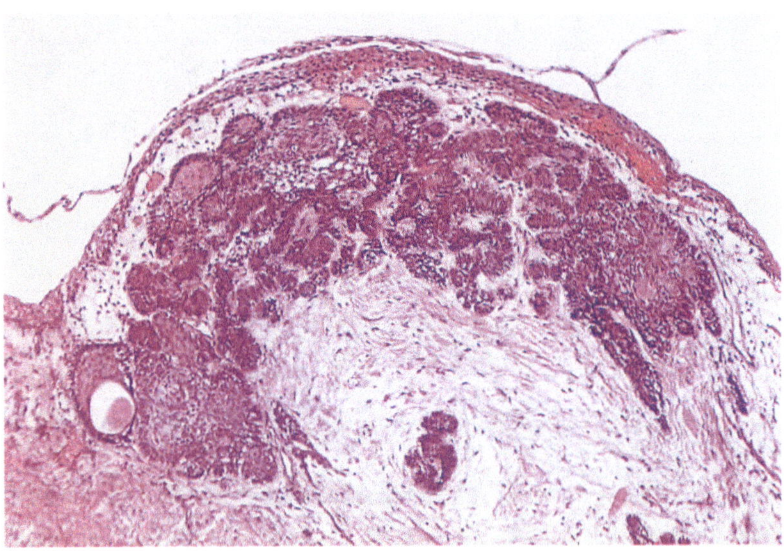

**Fig. 20.** *Ameloblastoma.* Tumour developing in wall of a dentigerous cyst. ×80

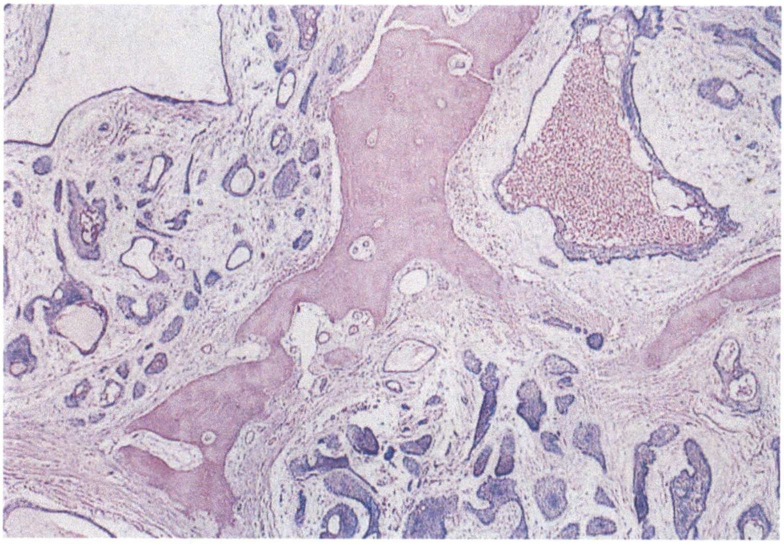

**Fig. 21.** *Ameloblastoma, follicular.* Typical pattern of extension through cancellous bone. ×32

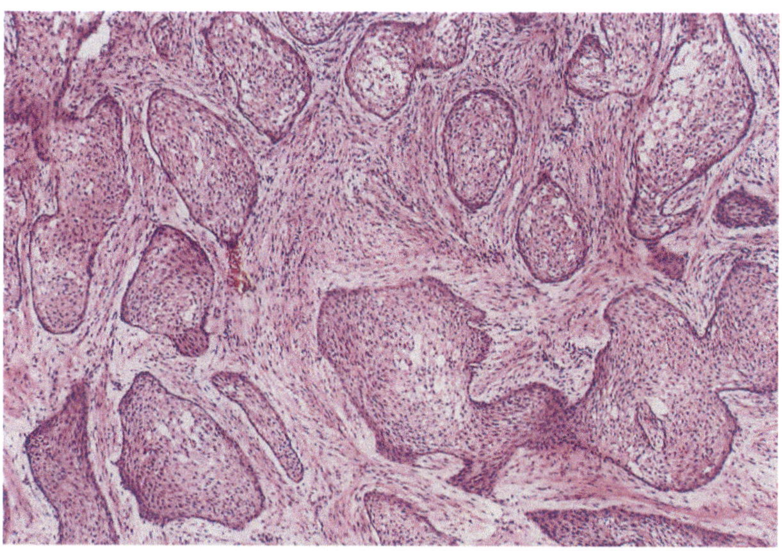

**Fig. 22.** *Squamous odontogenic tumour.* Islands of squamous epithelial cells, with no columnar cells at the periphery. ×50

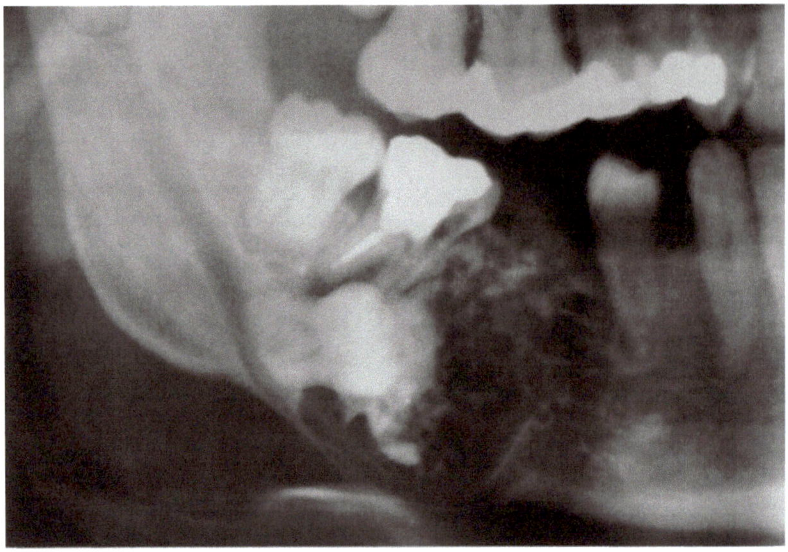

**Fig. 23.** *Calcifying epithelial odontogenic tumour,* mandible. Tumour shows patchy mineralization within radiolucent area next to crown of the embedded molar

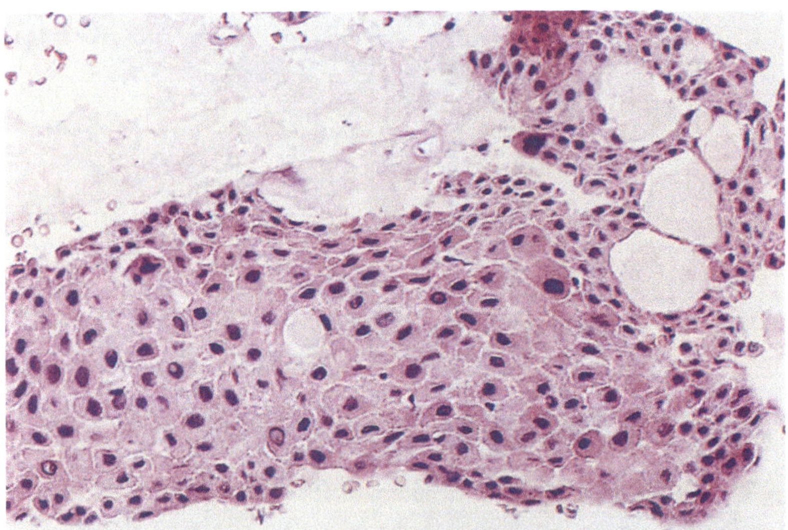

**Fig. 24.** *Calcifying epithelial odontogenic tumour.* Polyhedral cells with intercellular bridges and some nuclear pleomorphism. ×200

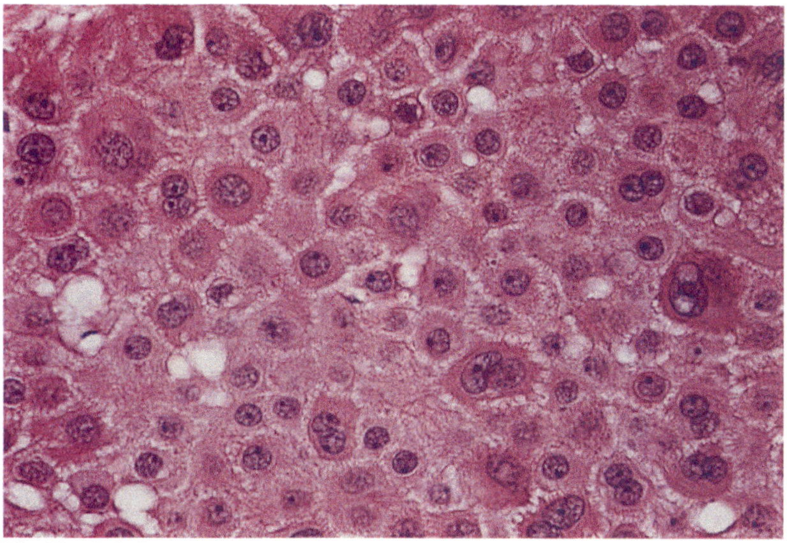

**Fig. 25.** *Calcifying epithelial odontogenic tumour.* Marked cellular and nuclear pleomorphism. ×510

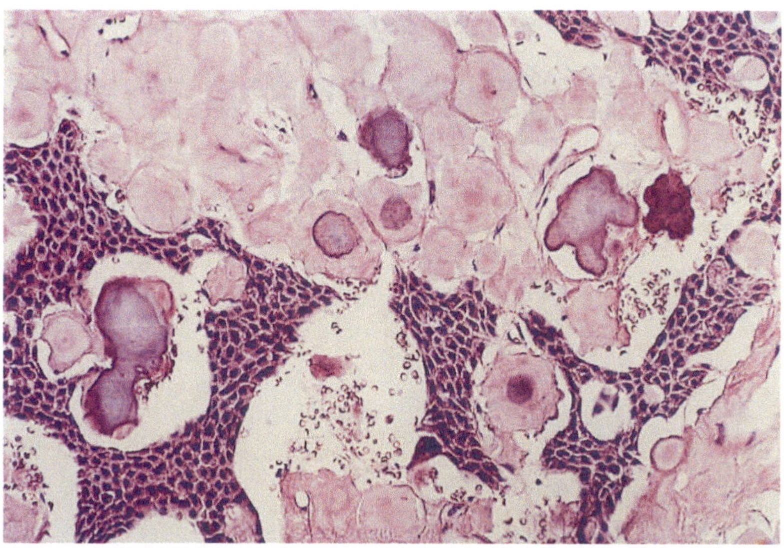

**Fig. 26.** *Calcifying epithelial odontogenic tumour.* Abundant rounded masses of amyloid-like material within the tumour. Some are calcified. ×160

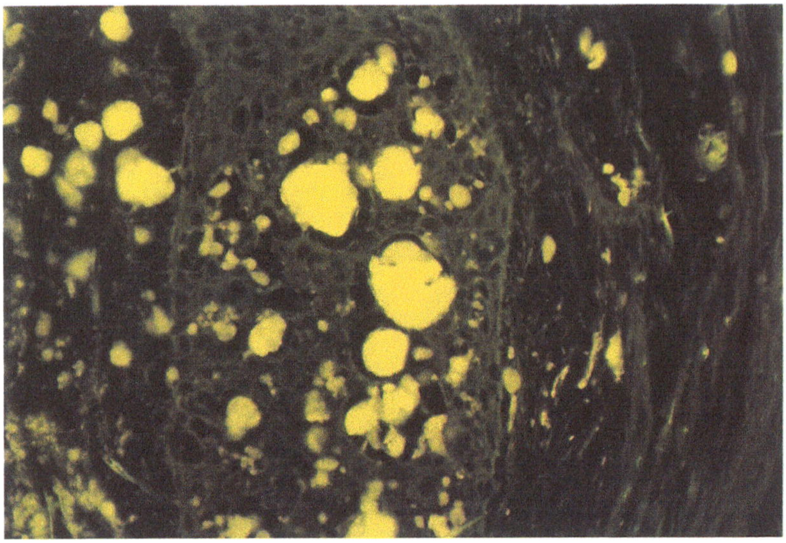

**Fig. 27.** *Calcifying epithelial odontogenic tumour.* Fluorescence of amyloid-like material stained with thioflavine T. × 160

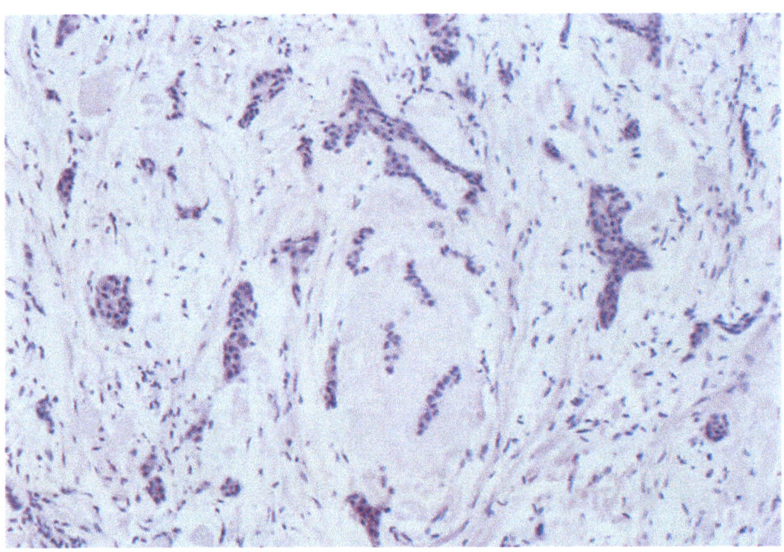

**Fig. 28.** *Peripheral calcifying epithelial odontogenic tumour.* Generally this tumour appears less active than intraosseous forms. × 140

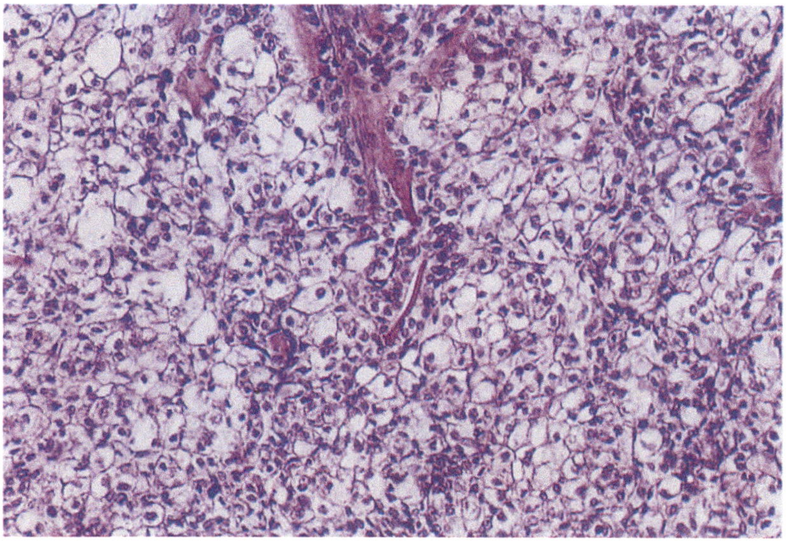

**Fig. 29.** *Clear cell odontogenic tumour.* Sheets of clear cells, some with a faintly stippled cytoplasm. ×200

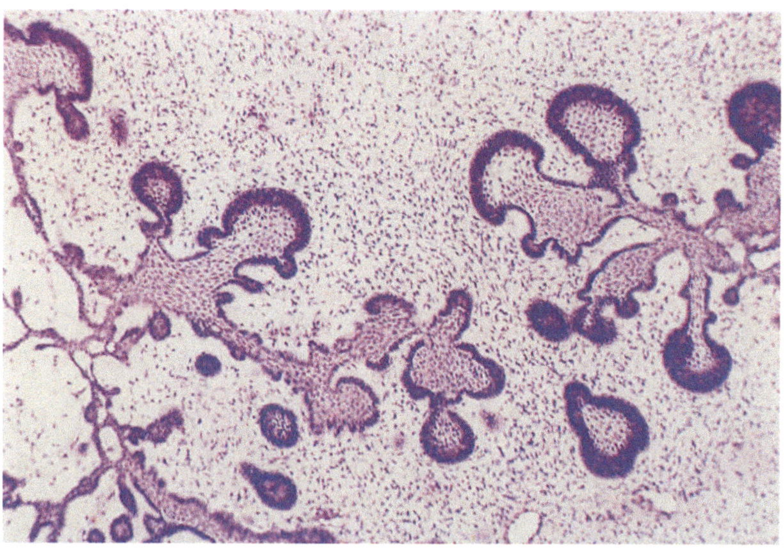

**Fig. 30.** *Ameloblastic fibroma.* Proliferating odontogenic epithelium and cell-rich mesenchyme. ×80

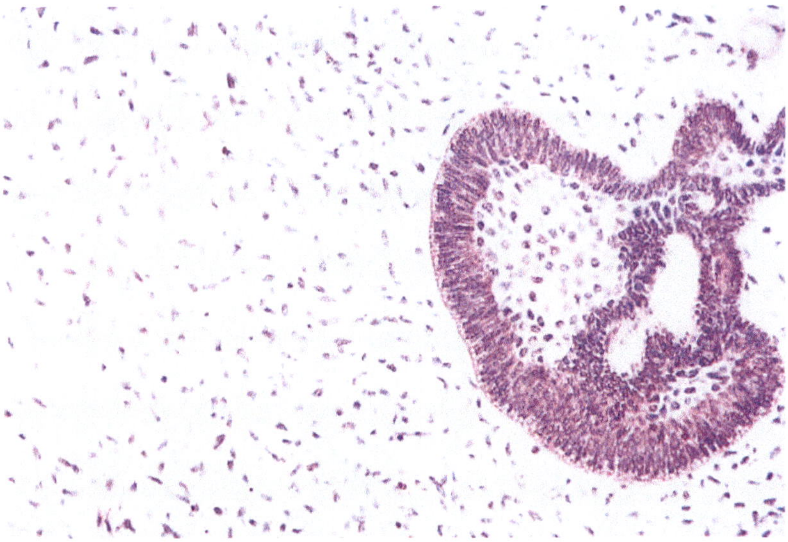

**Fig. 31.** *Ameloblastic fibroma.* The cell-rich mesenchymal component resembles dental papilla (see Fig. 2b). ×200

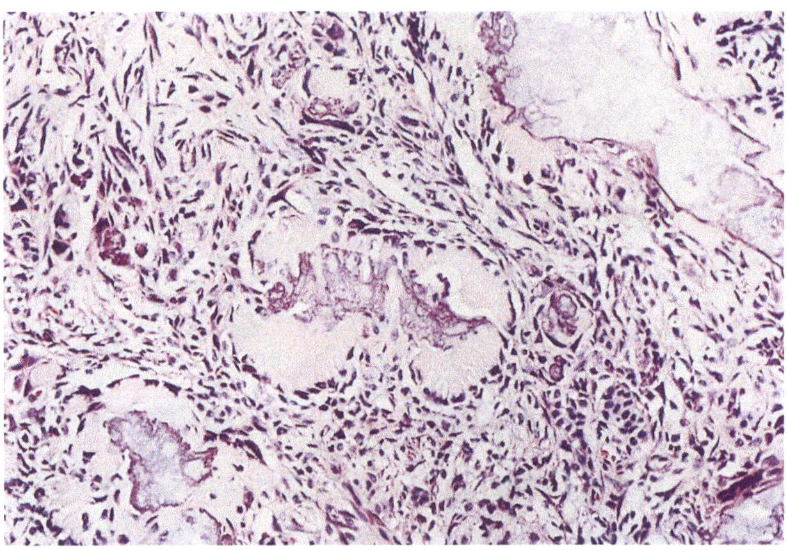

**Fig. 32.** *Ameloblastic fibrodentinoma.* Islands of dysplastic and poorly mineralized dentine. ×200

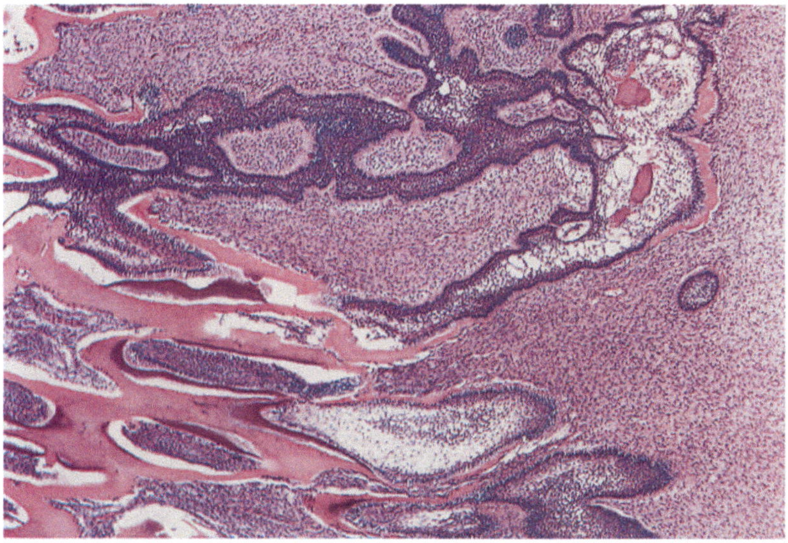

**Fig. 33.** *Ameloblastic fibro-odontoma.* Odontogenic epithelium and cell-rich mesenchyme at *upper right;* dentine (acidophilic) and enamel (basophilic) at *lower left.* ×32

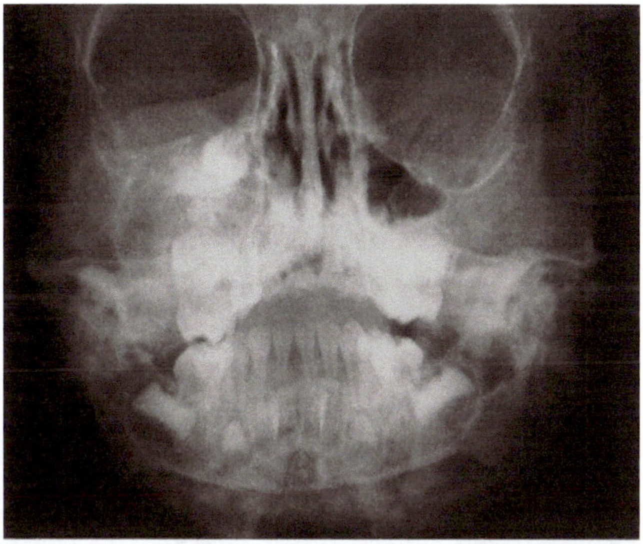

**Fig. 34.** *Ameloblastic fibro-odontoma,* right maxilla. Lesion extends to orbital floor and contains radiopaque areas of varying size

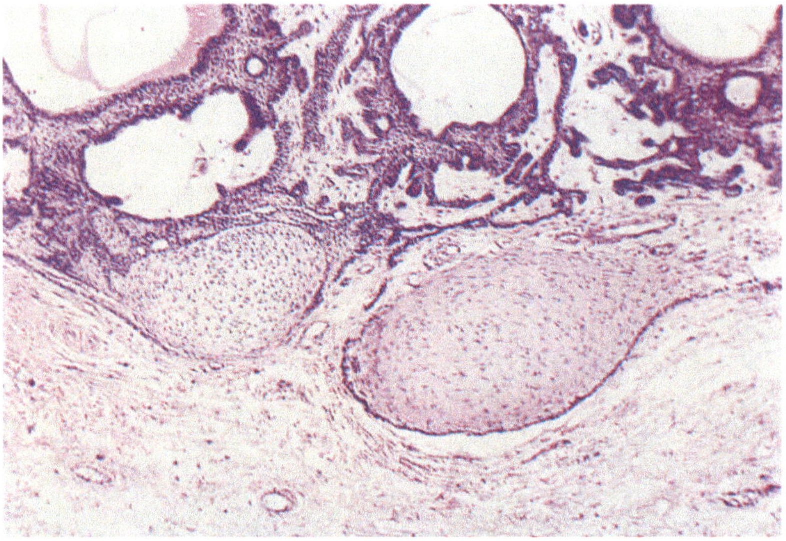

**Fig. 35.** *Odontoameloblastoma.* Two ovoid masses of odontogenic mesenchyme lie next to epithelium showing plexiform ameloblastoma pattern. ×80

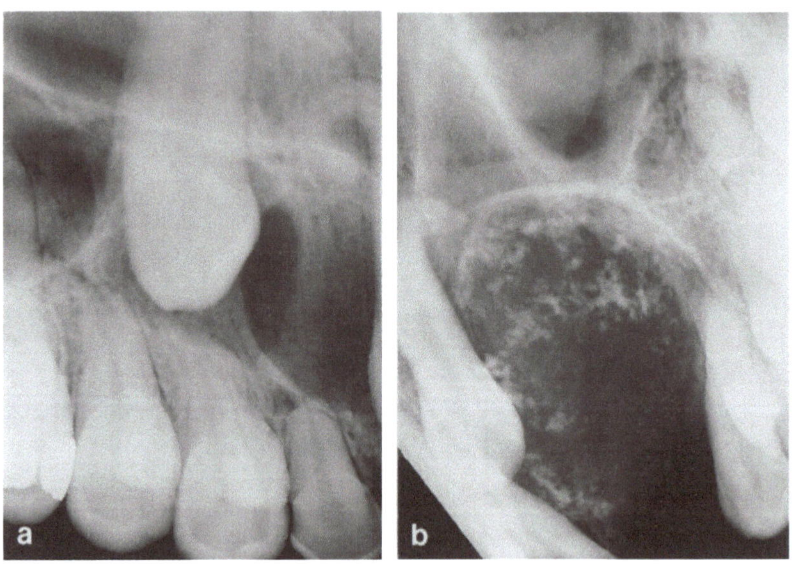


**Fig. 36 a, b.** *Adenomatoid odontogenic tumour.* **a** Radiolucent lesion associated with crown of embedded tooth. **b** Similar lesion, but with areas of mineralization.

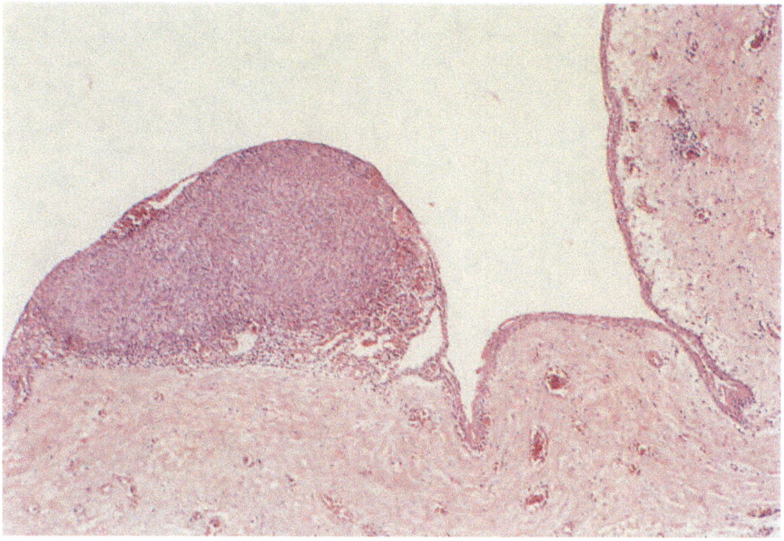

**Fig. 37.** *Adenomatoid odontogenic tumour.* Focus of tumour forming part of cyst wall. ×50

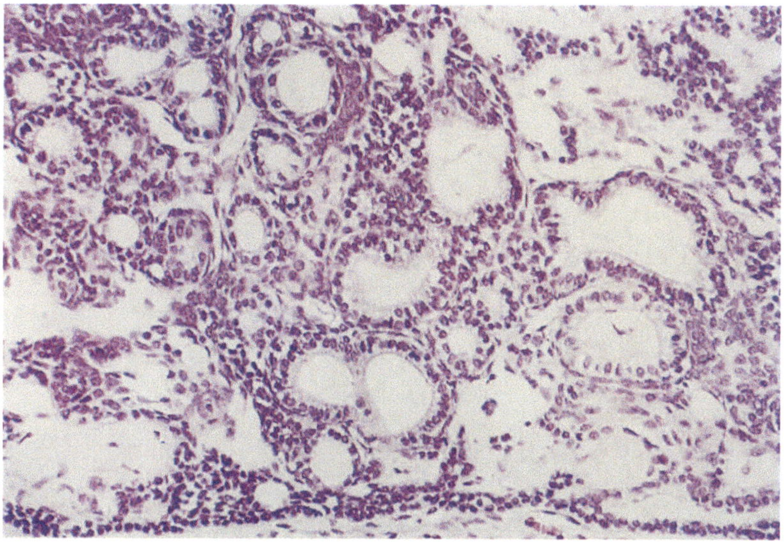

**Fig. 38.** *Adenomatoid odontogenic tumour.* The epithelium shows multiple duct-like structures. ×200

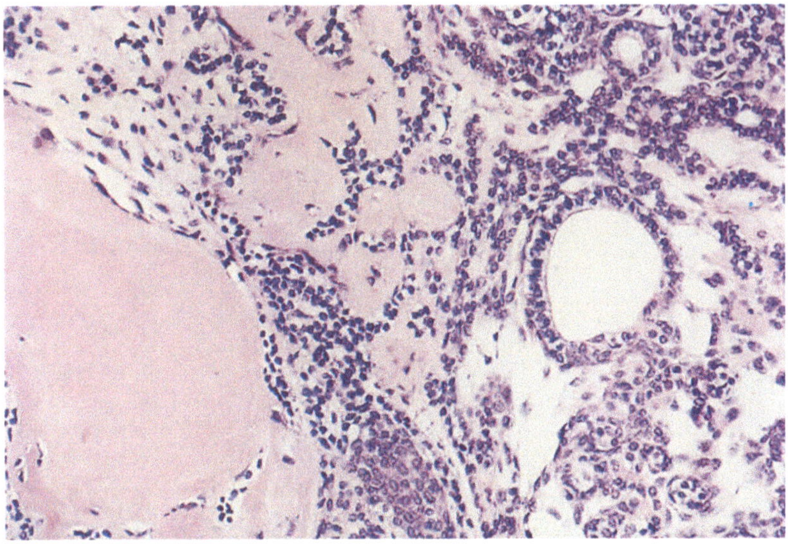

**Fig. 39.** *Adenomatoid odontogenic tumour.* Duct-like epithelial structures and sheets of acidophilic material resembling dysplastic dentine. ×200

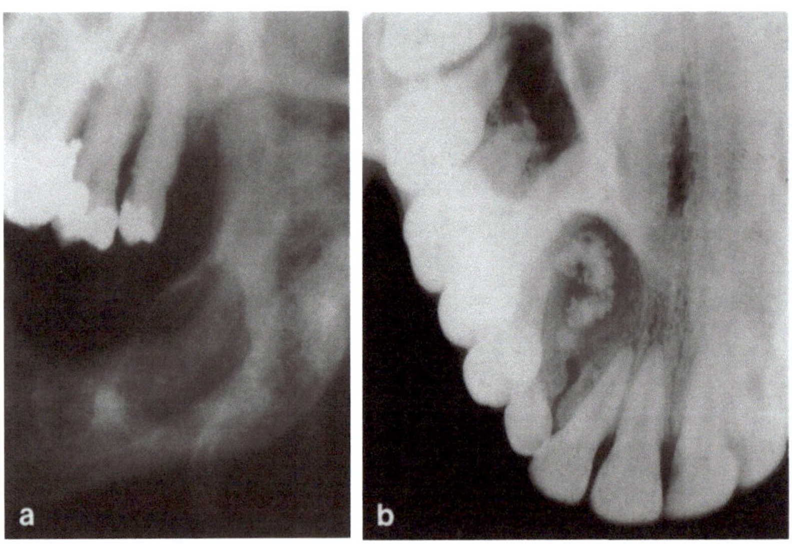


**Fig. 40 a, b.** *Calcifying odontogenic cyst.* **a** Mandibular lesion. **b** Maxillary lesion with considerable mineralization

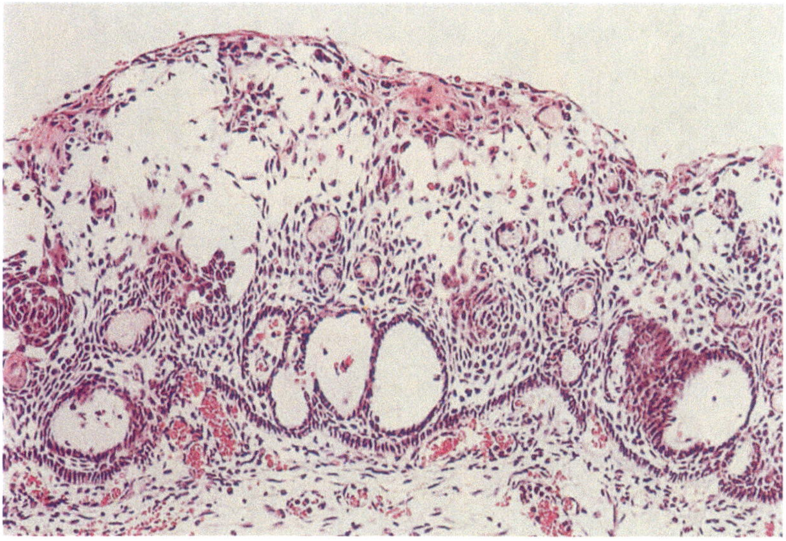

**Fig. 41.** *Calcifying odontogenic cyst.* Cyst lining shows columnar basal cells and upper layers resembling stellate reticulum but including scattered ghost cells. ×200

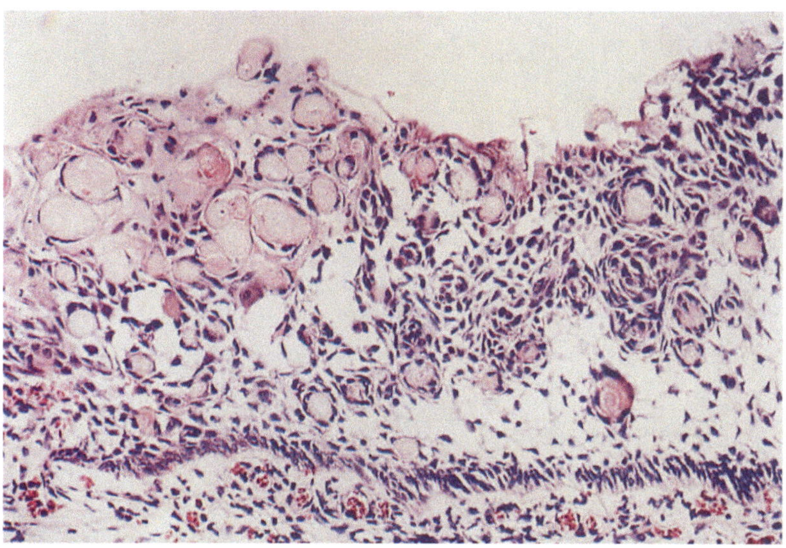

**Fig. 42.** *Calcifying odontogenic cyst.* Ghost cells lying individually and in small groups. ×200

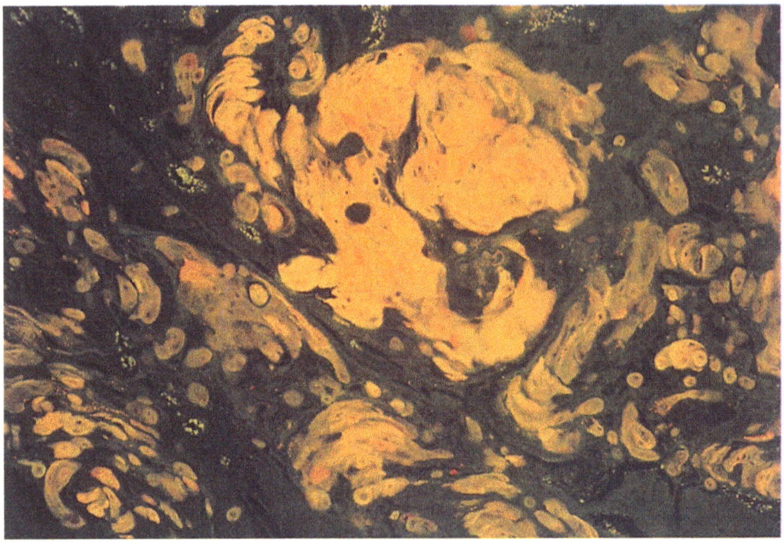

**Fig. 43.** *Calcifying odontogenic cyst.* Ghost cells showing fluorescence after staining with rhodamine B. ×130

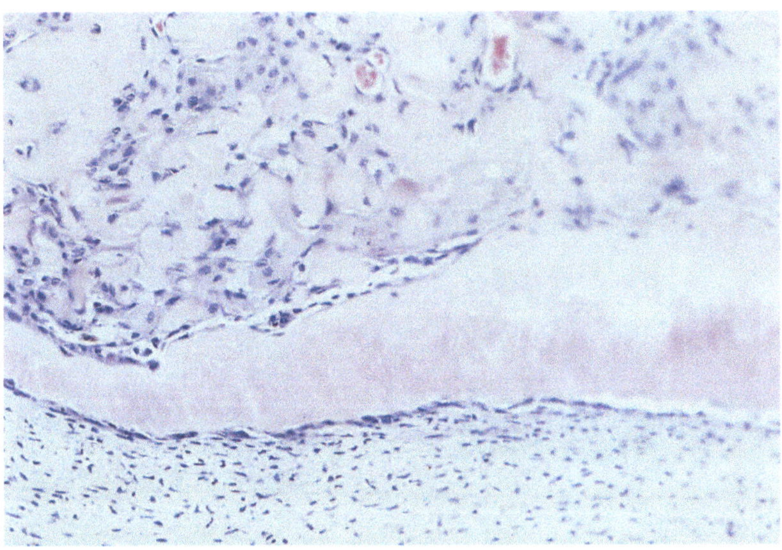

**Fig. 44.** *Calcifying odontogenic cyst.* A band of dentine has been formed by odontogenic mesenchyme lying beneath the epithelium. ×130

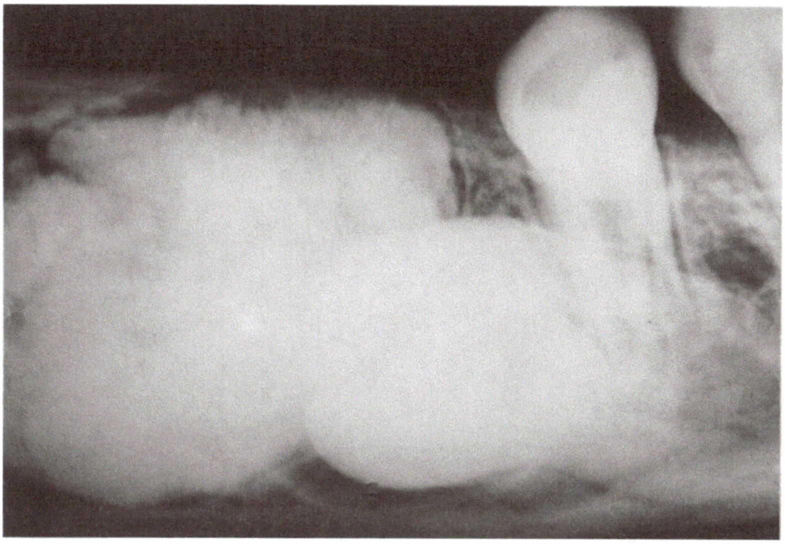

**Fig. 45.** *Complex odontoma.* Dense radiopaque mass lying next to an impacted molar

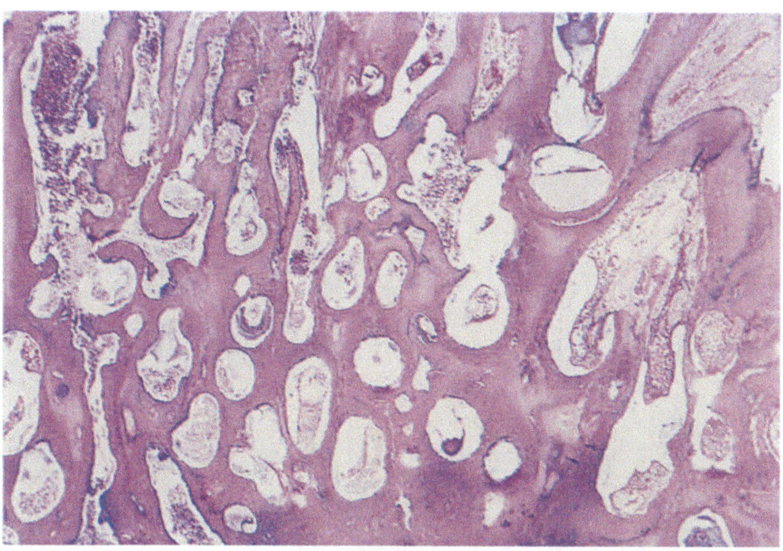

**Fig. 46.** *Complex odontoma.* Disordered mixture of dental tissues. ×32

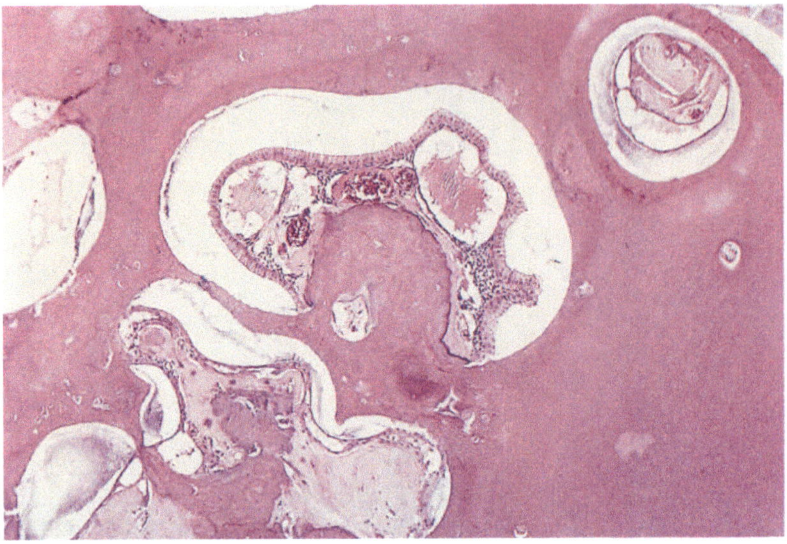

**Fig. 47.** *Complex odontoma.* Odontogenic epithelium is still identifiable in spaces within dentine. Before demineralization, gaps between epithelium and dentine contained enamel. ×80

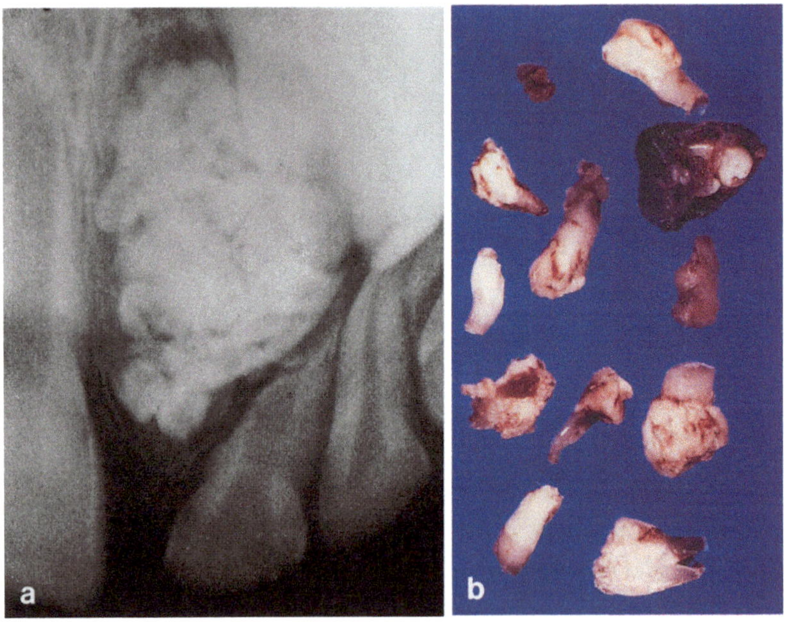


**Fig. 48 a, b.** *Compound odontoma.* **a** Lesion in maxillary incisor region. **b** Operation specimen: the lesion is composed of many small denticles

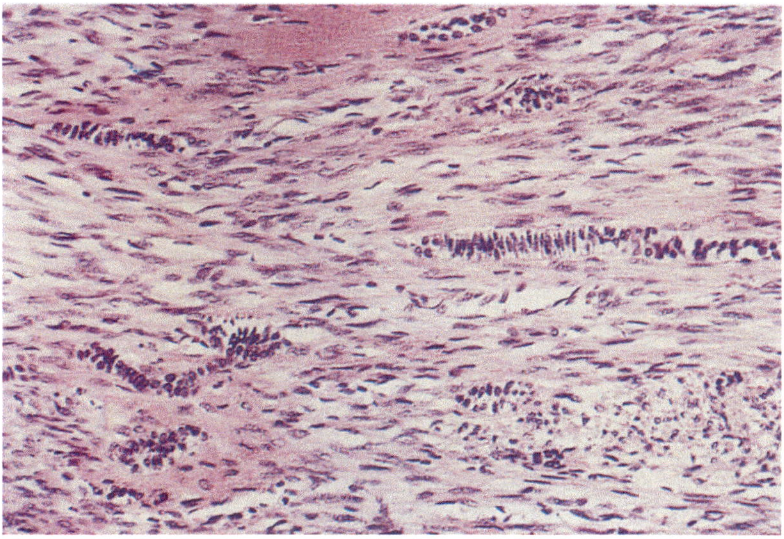

**Fig. 49.** *Odontogenic fibroma.* Cellular fibroblastic tissue containing strands of odontogenic epithelium. ×200

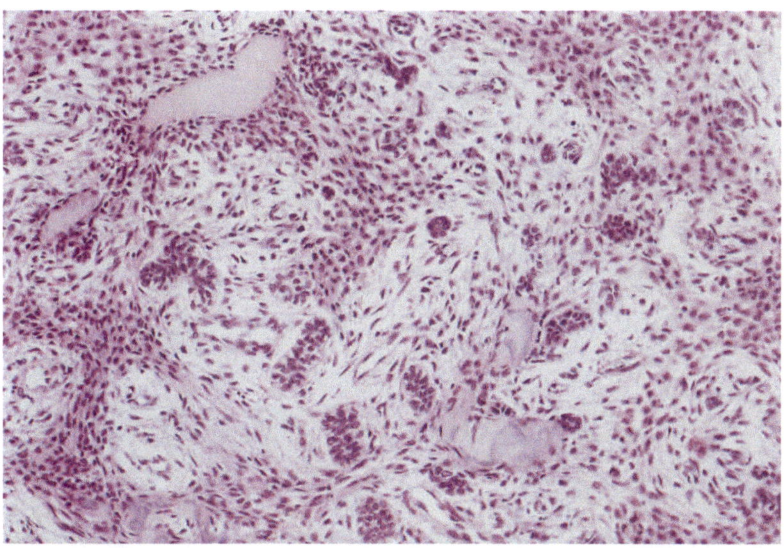

**Fig. 50.** *Odontogenic fibroma.* Fibrous tissue containing epithelium and islands of dysplastic cementum or bone. ×180

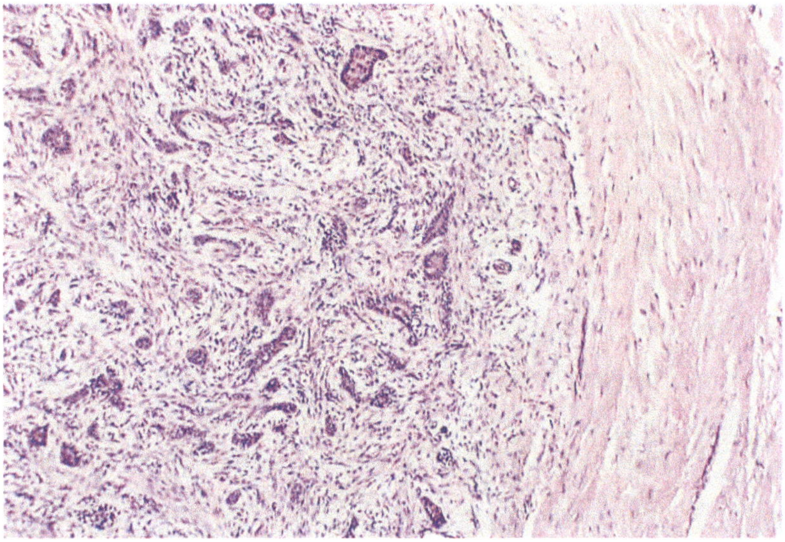

**Fig. 51.** *Odontogenic fibroma.* Peripheral lesion with much epithelium. ×80

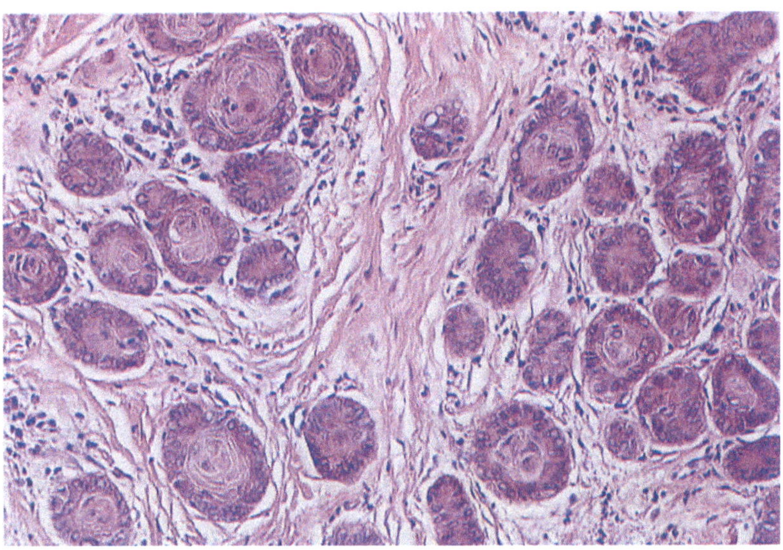

**Fig. 52.** *Odontogenic gingival epithelial hamartoma.* Epithelium lies in mature fibrous tissue. ×200

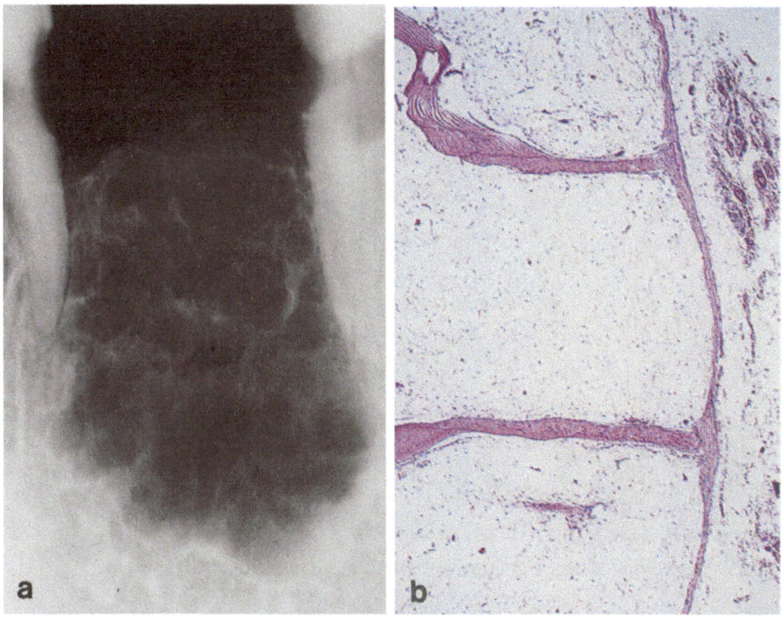

**Fig. 53 a, b.** *Myxoma.* **a** Mandibular lesion showing typical 'soap-bubble' appearance. **b** Tumour extending through bone. ×32

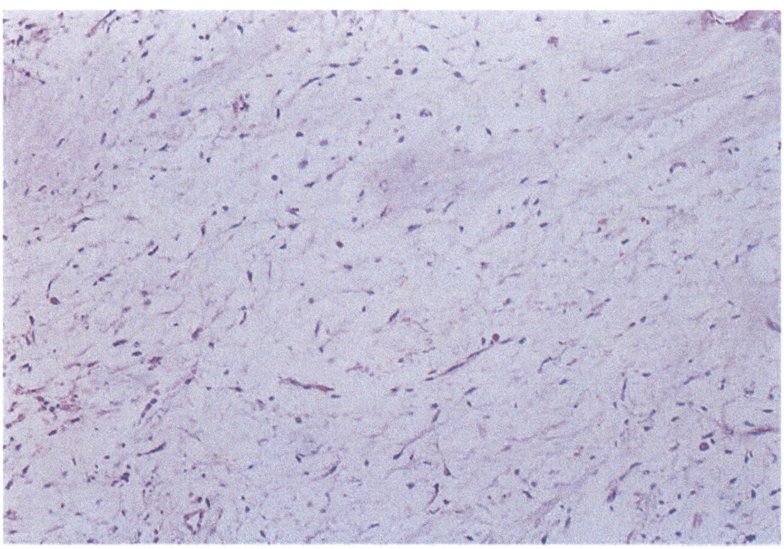

**Fig. 54.** *Myxoma.* ×32

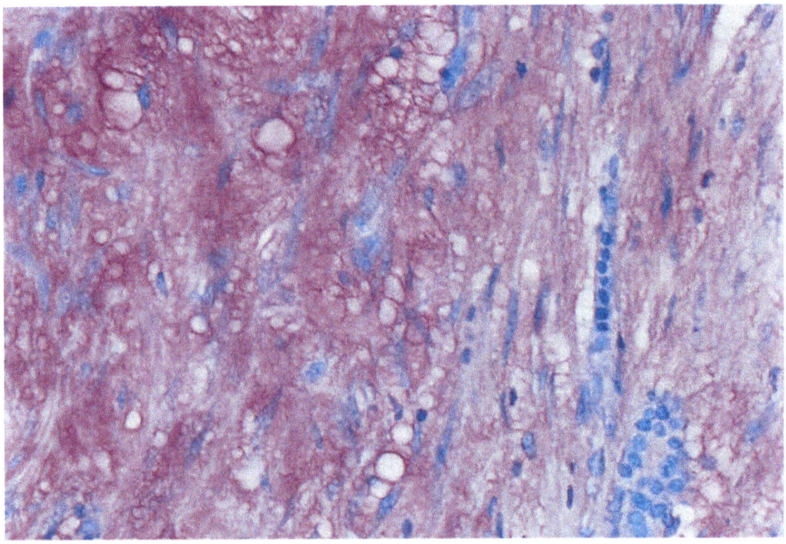

**Fig. 55.** *Myxoma.* Mucoid ground substance. Alcian blue. ×160

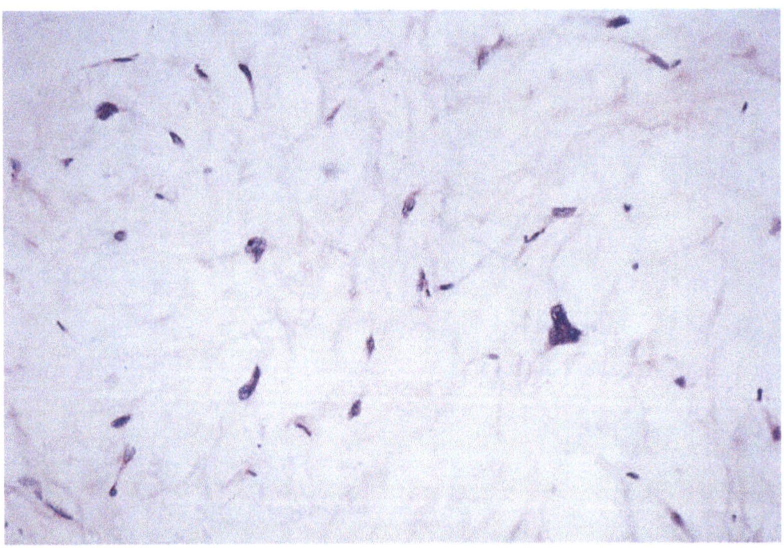

**Fig. 56.** *Myxoma.* Widely separated cells with abundant mucoid ground substance. Some cells show nuclear atypia. ×200

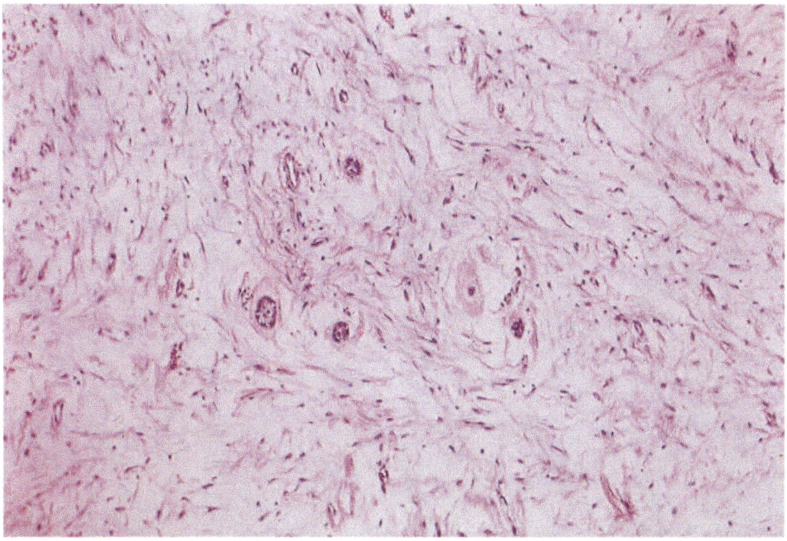

**Fig. 57.** Dental follicle. Thickened follicle from an unerupted tooth, simulating a myxoma. ×80

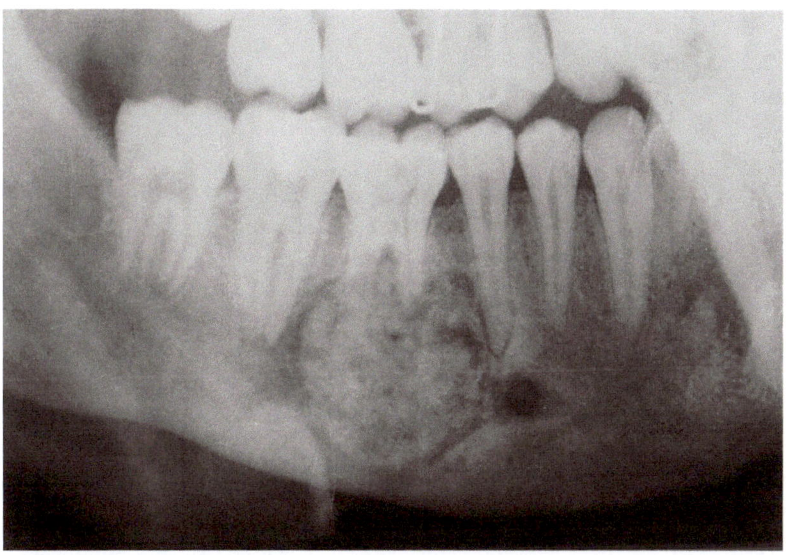

**Fig. 58.** *Benign cementoblastoma.* Rounded mass related to roots of mandibular first permanent molar

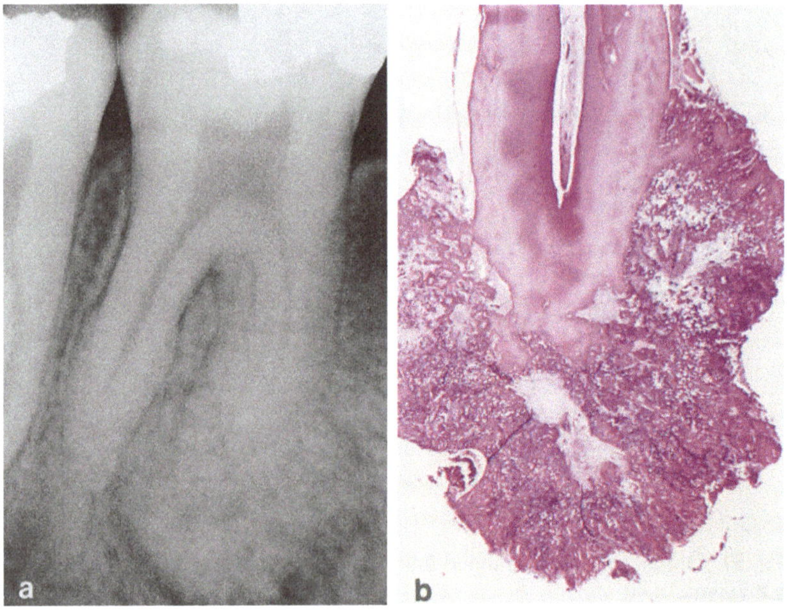

**Fig. 59 a, b.** *Benign cementoblastoma.* **a** Mass attached to anterior root of mandibular molar. **b** Same lesion; partial resorption of root and fusion of tumour to root surface. ×16

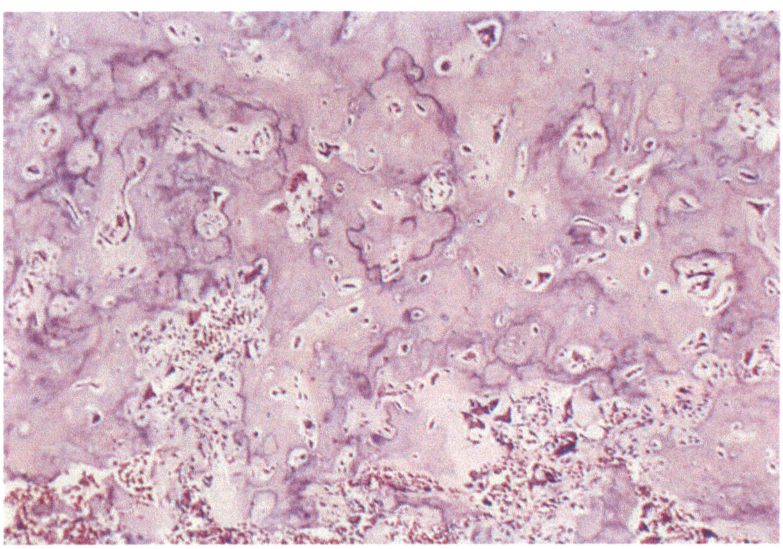

**Fig. 60.** *Benign cementoblastoma.* Basophilic reversal lines. ×80

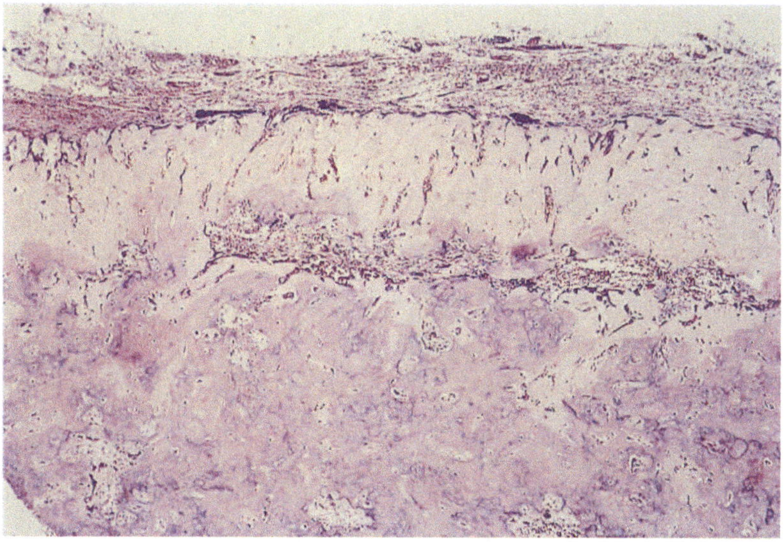

**Fig. 61.** *Benign cementoblastoma.* Peripheral unmineralized zone with no remodelling; remodelling in underlying mineralized tissue. ×32

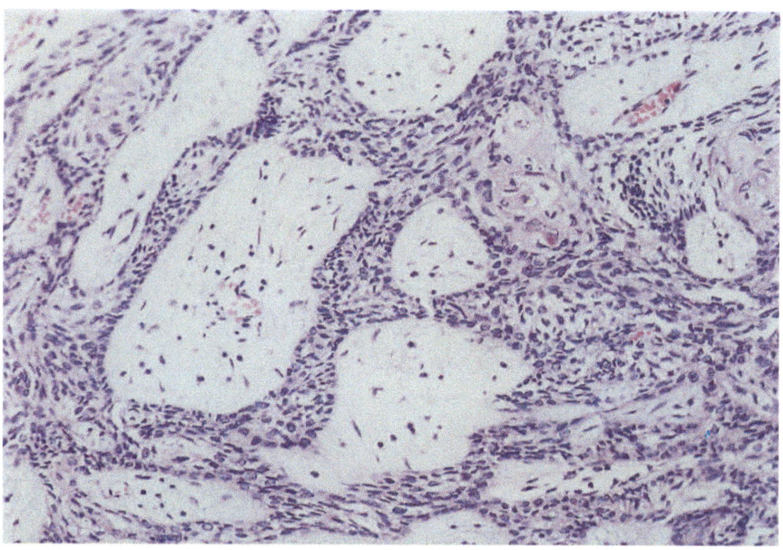

**Fig. 62.** *Malignant ameloblastoma.* ×160

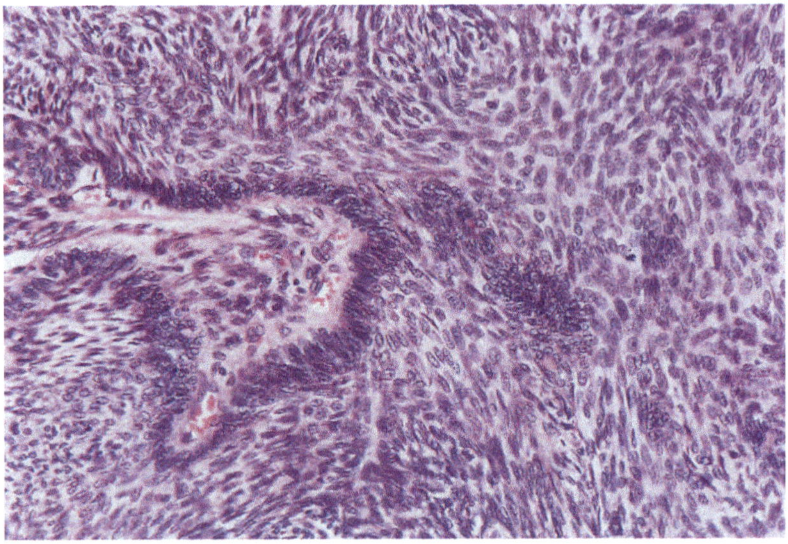

**Fig. 63.** *Malignant ameloblastoma.* Crowded epithelial cells and mitotic activity. ×200

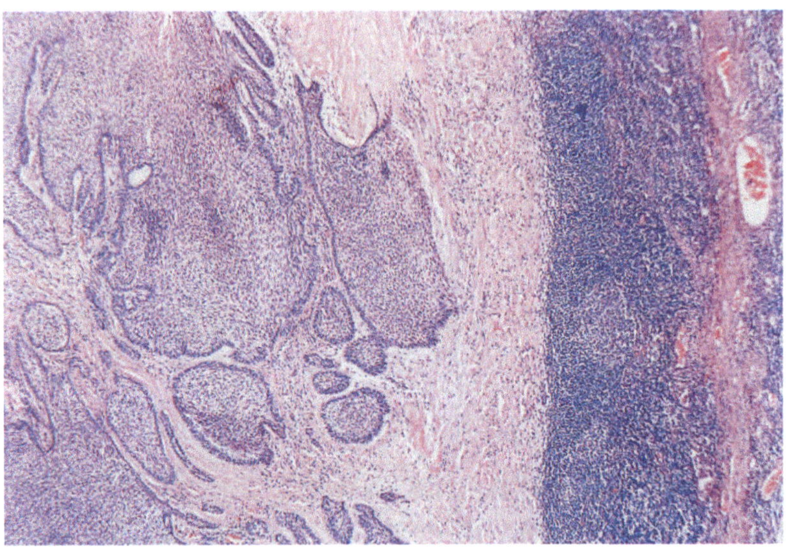

**Fig. 64.** *Malignant ameloblastoma.* Same patient as Figs. 62 and 63. Tumour in regional lymph node. ×45

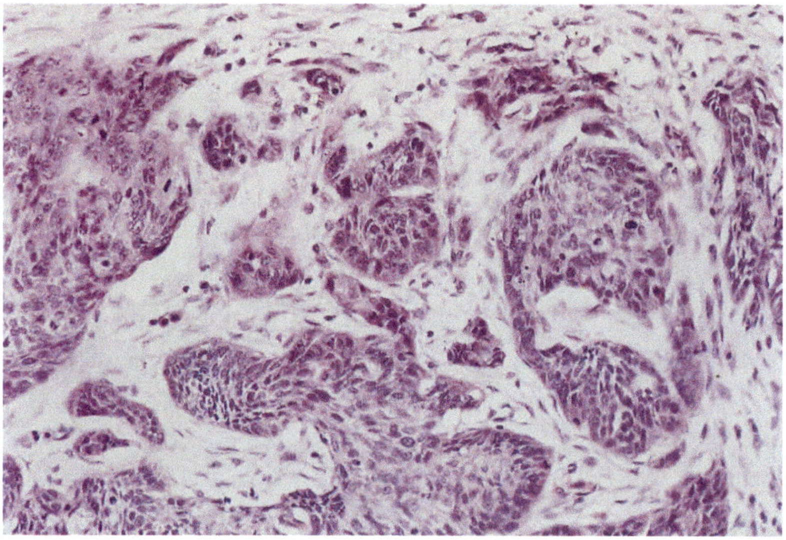

**Fig. 65.** *Primary intraosseous carcinoma.* Intraosseous squamous cell carcinoma. No connection to surface epithelium or evidence of tumour elsewhere. ×200

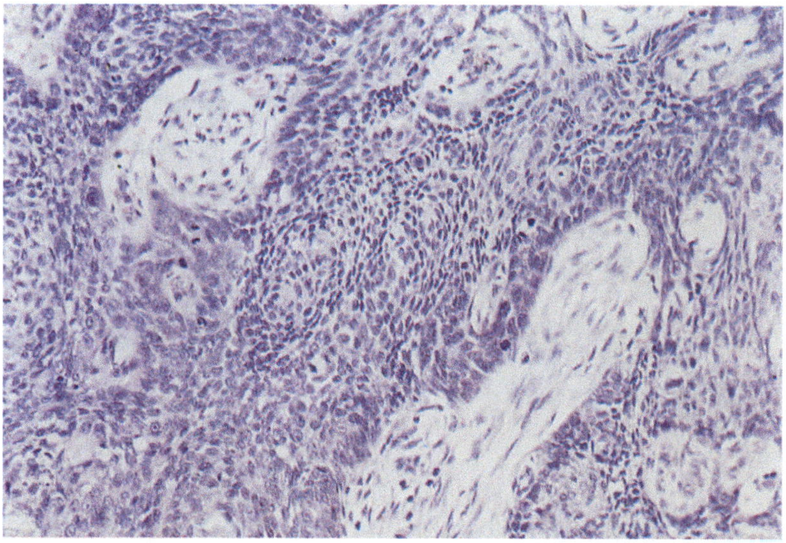

**Fig. 66.** *Primary intraosseous carcinoma.* Tumour pattern suggests origin from odontogenic epithelium. ×200

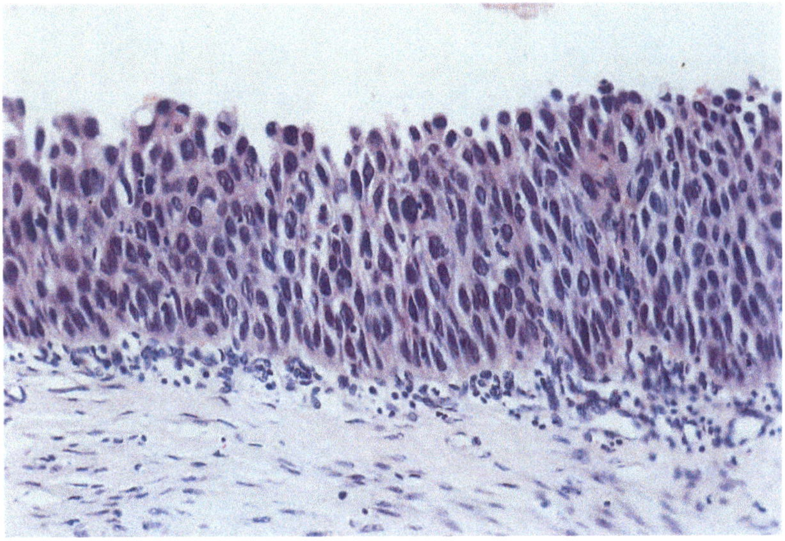

**Fig. 67.** *Epithelial dysplasia* in cyst wall. × 200

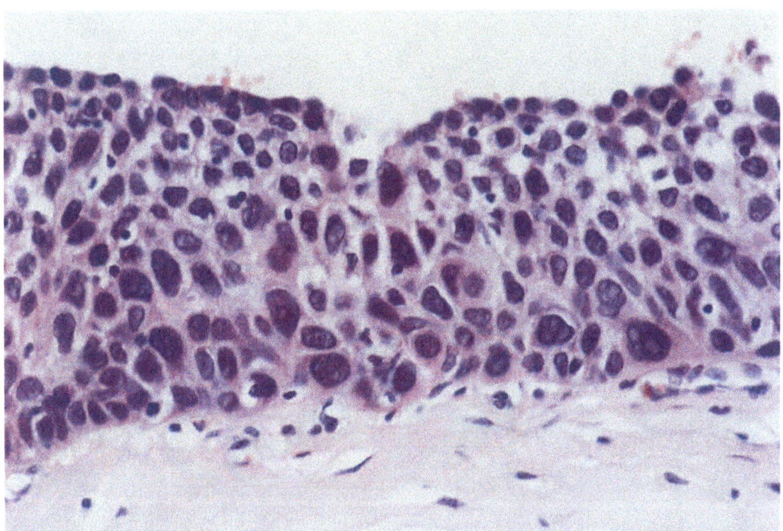

**Fig. 68.** *Epithelial dysplasia* in cyst wall. × 200

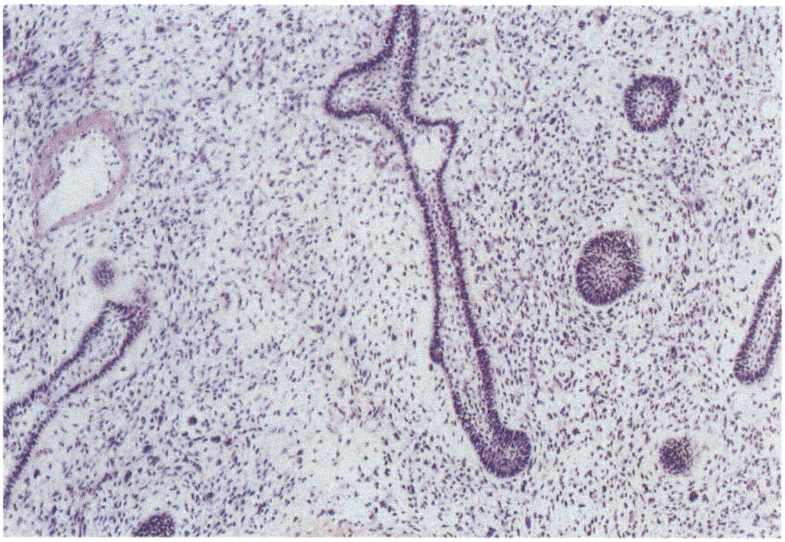

**Fig. 69.** *Ameloblastic fibrosarcoma.* Odontogenic epithelium lying in richly cellular odontogenic mesenchyme. ×80

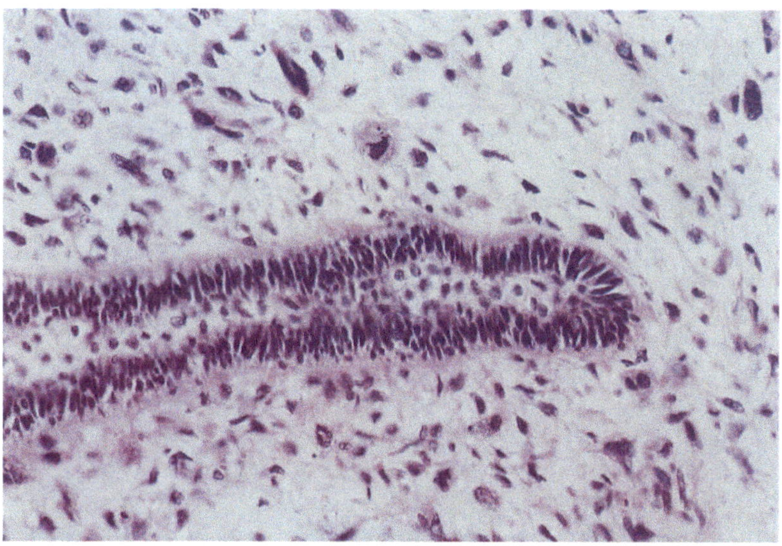

**Fig. 70.** *Ameloblastic fibrosarcoma.* Malignant features in mesenchymal component. ×320

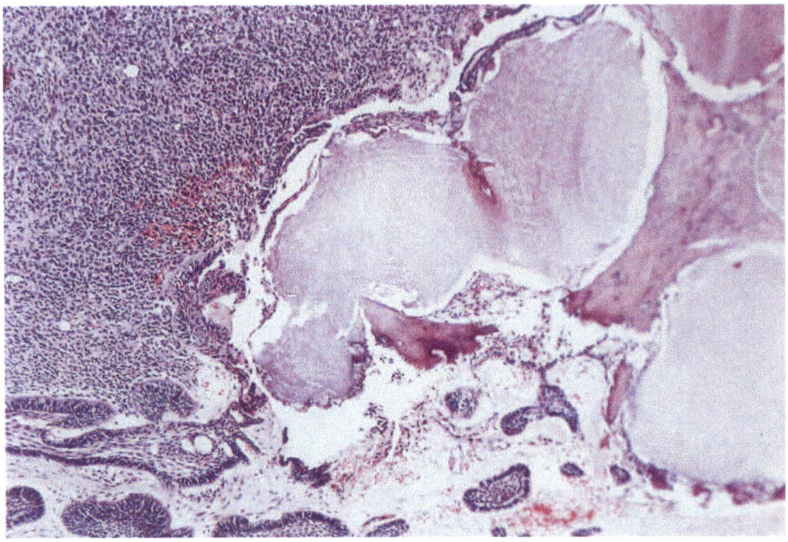

**Fig. 71.** *Ameloblastic fibro-odontosarcoma.* Tumour includes enamel and dysplastic dentine. ×65

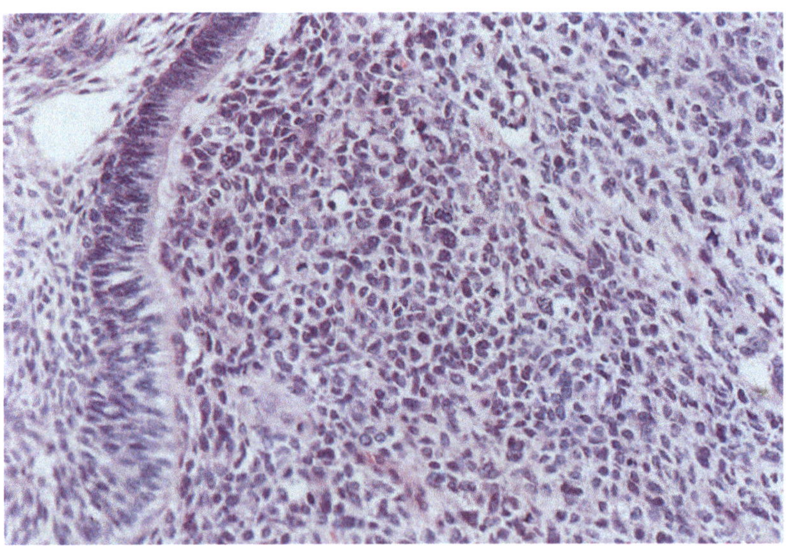

**Fig. 72.** *Ameloblastic fibro-odontosarcoma.* Pleomorphism in mesenchymal component. ×200

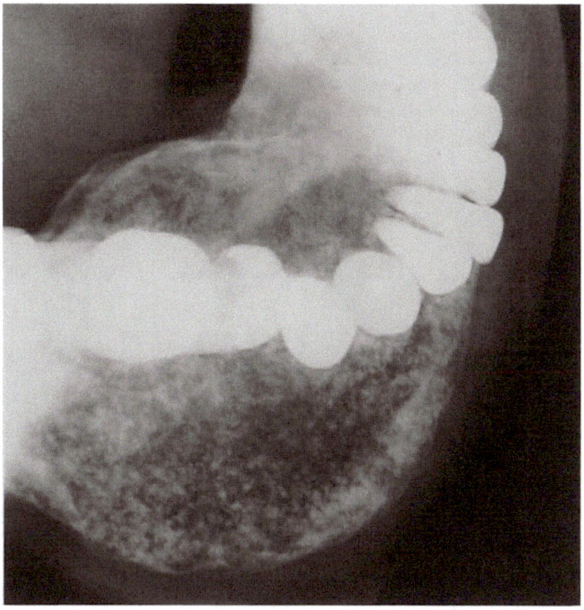

**Fig. 73.** *Cemento-ossifying fibroma,* mandible. Well-defined lesion with patchy mineralization

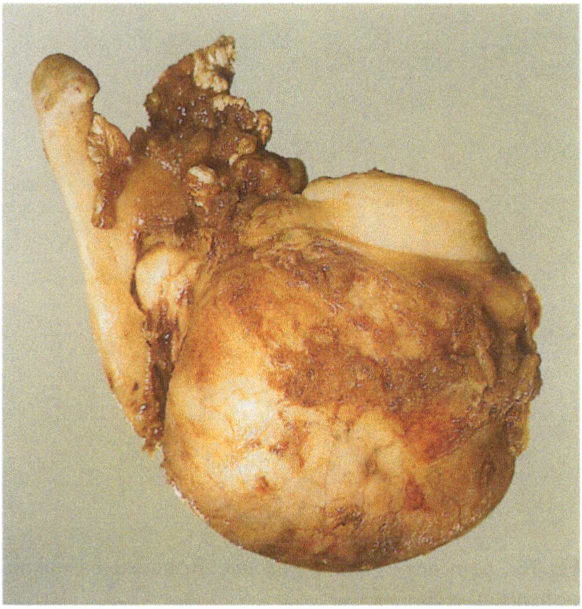

**Fig. 74.** *Cemento-ossifying fibroma,* mandible. The tumour has a smooth surface and is well demarcated from the bone

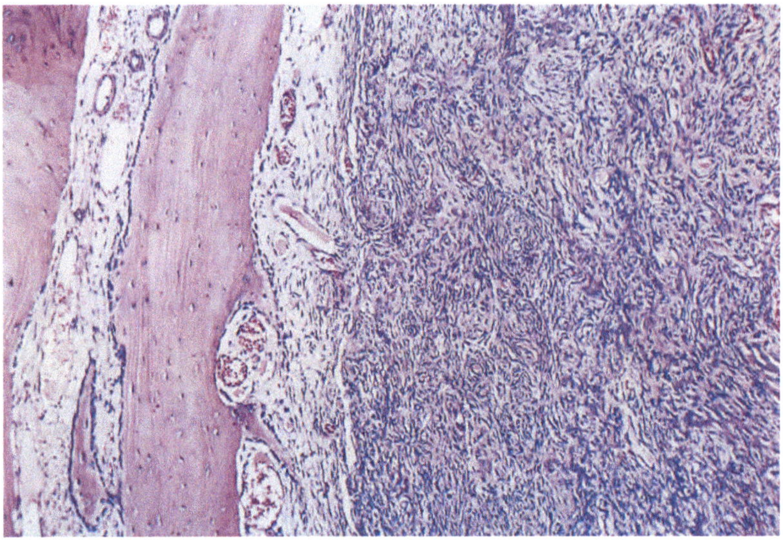

**Fig. 75.** *Cemento-ossifying fibroma.* Demarcation of lesion from adjacent bone. ×80

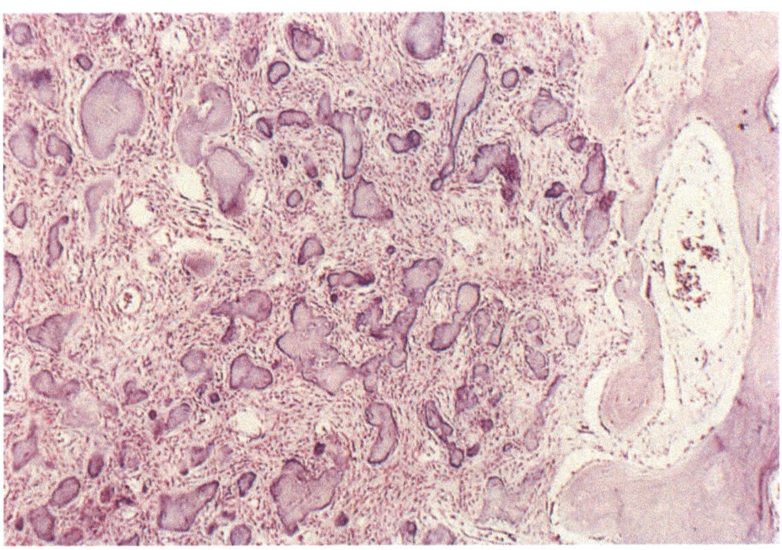

**Fig. 76.** *Cemento-ossifying fibroma.* Rounded basophilic masses resembling cementum. ×80

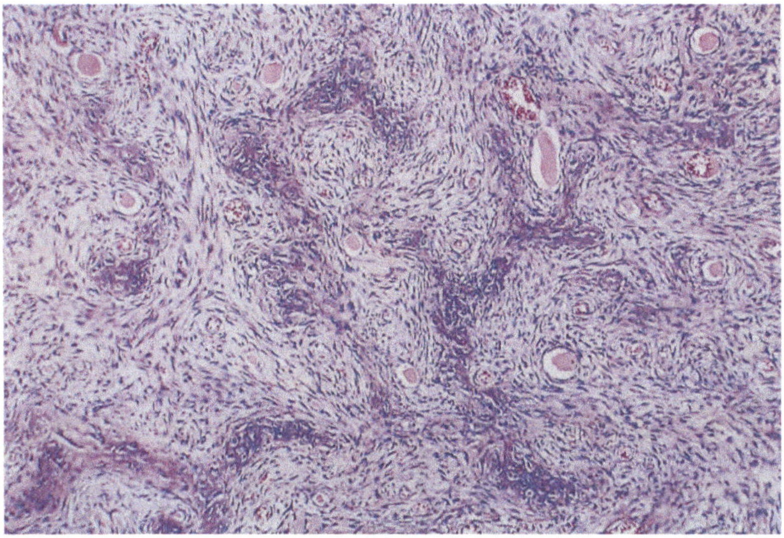

**Fig. 77.** *Cemento-ossifying fibroma.* Typical metaplastic bone. ×80

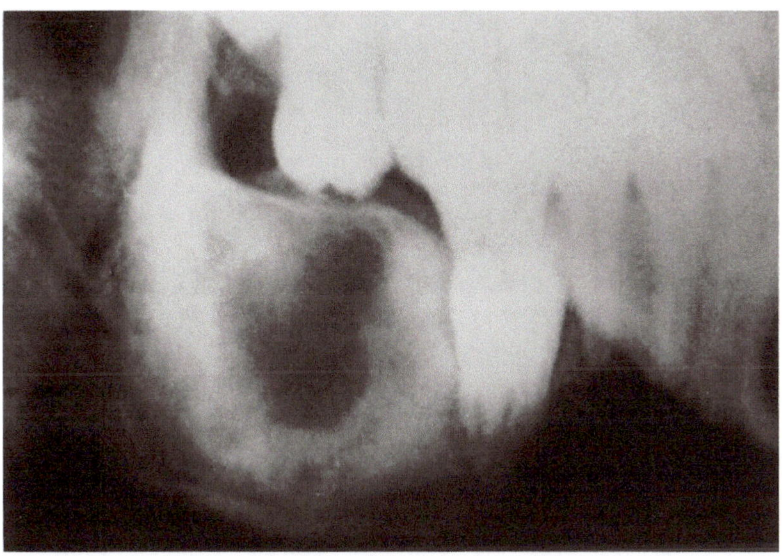

**Fig. 78.** *Fibrous dysplasia,* mandible. The lesion has ill-defined margins

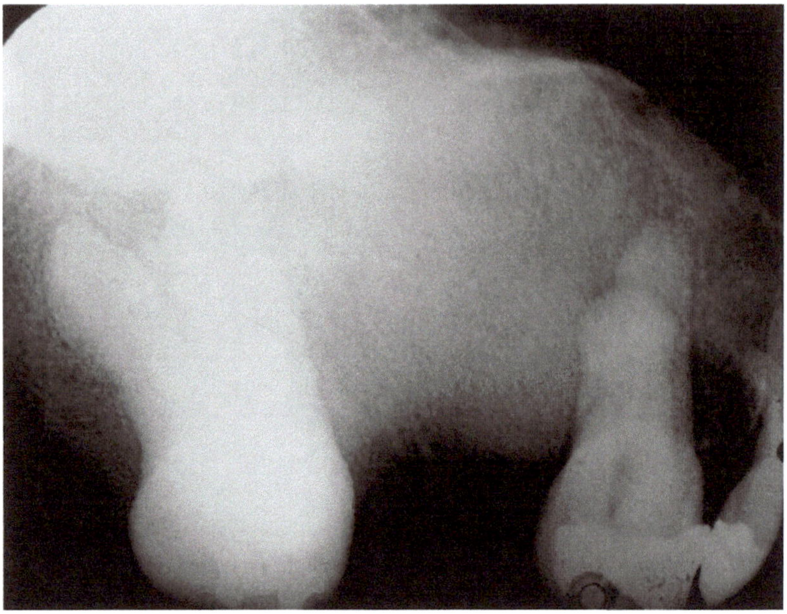

**Fig. 79.** *Fibrous dysplasia,* maxilla. 'Ground-glass' appearance. The lesion blends with the adjacent bone

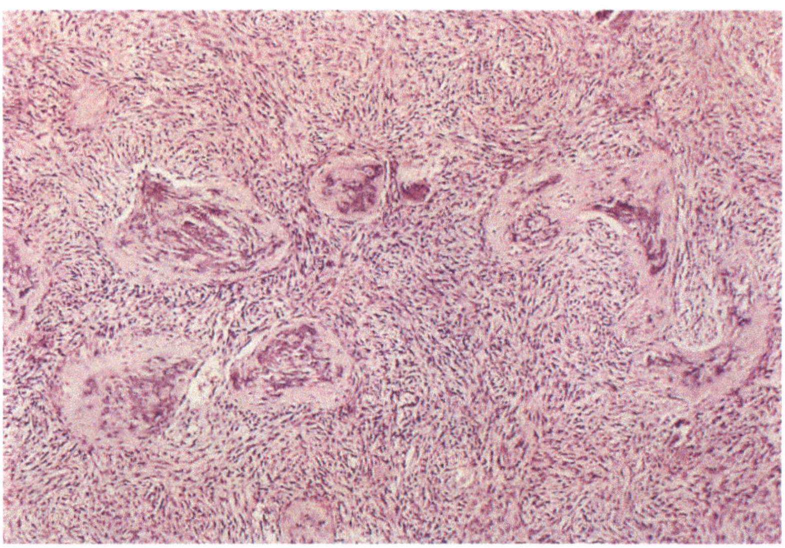

**Fig. 80.** *Fibrous dysplasia.* Richly cellular fibrous tissue with islands of metaplastic bone. ×80

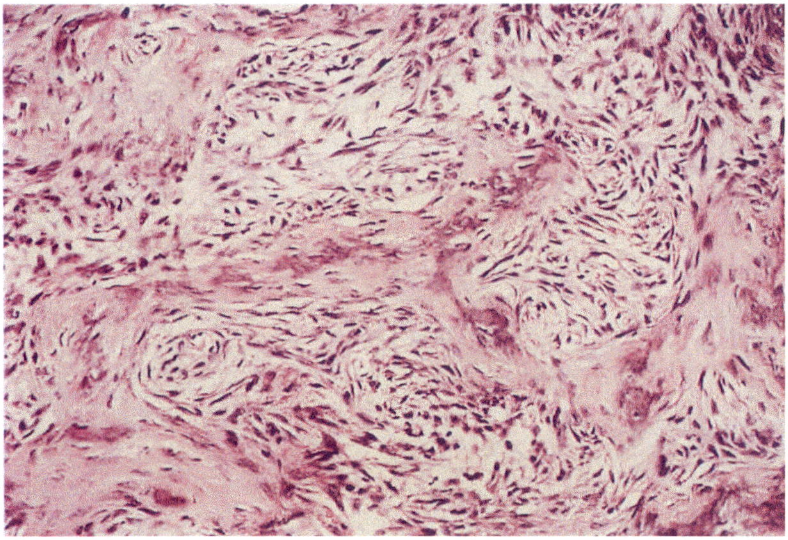

**Fig. 81.** *Fibrous dysplasia.* Trabeculae of metaplastic bone. ×200

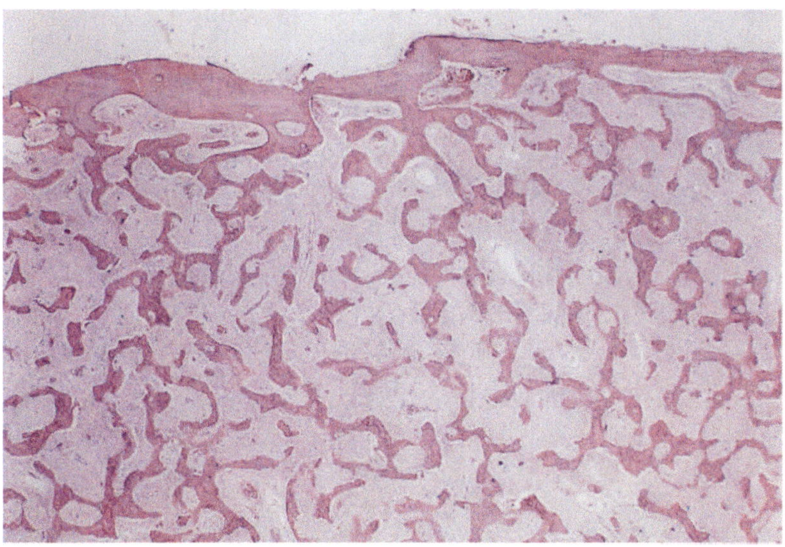

**Fig. 82.** *Fibrous dysplasia.* Lesional bone is fused to surrounding bone. ×20

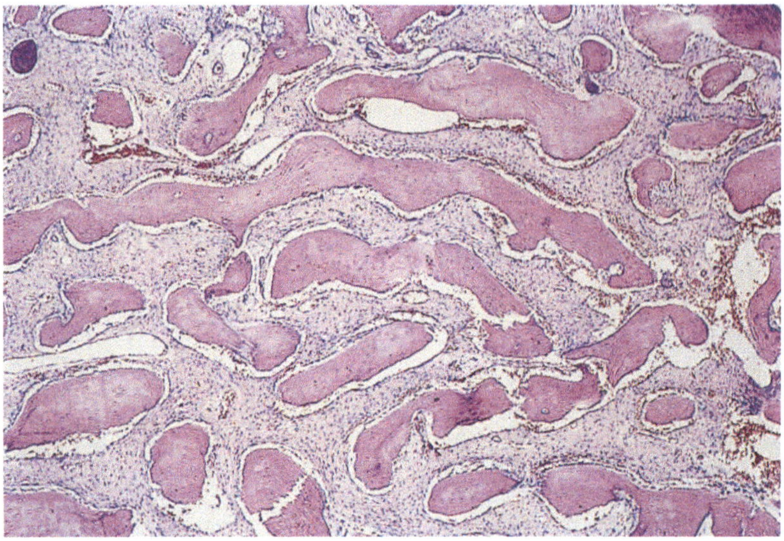

**Fig. 83.** *Fibrous dysplasia.* Old lesion; trabeculae of lamellar bone in moderately cellular fibrous stroma. ×32

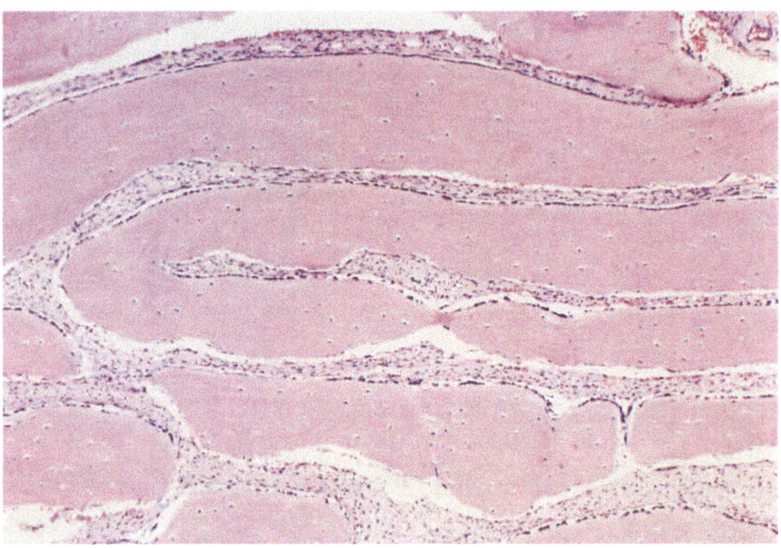

**Fig. 84.** *Fibrous dysplasia.* Old lesion; closely-placed parallel trabeculae of lamellar bone. ×80

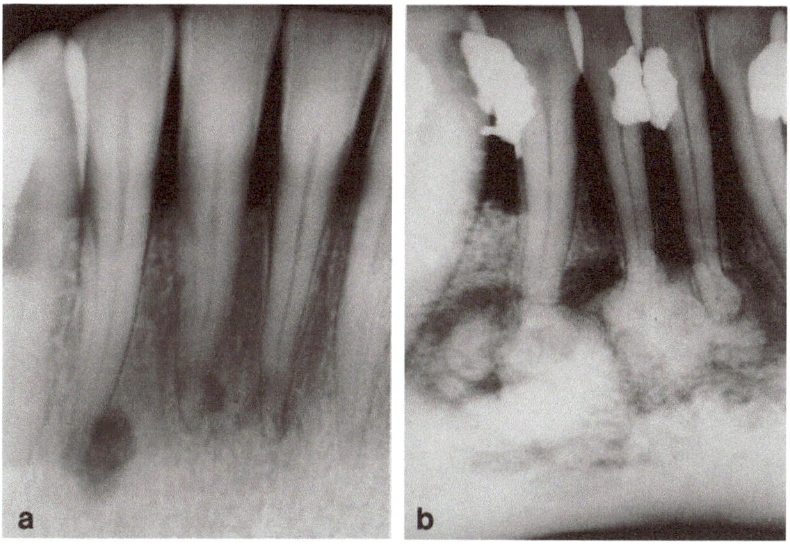


**Fig. 85 a, b.** *Periapical cemental dysplasia* **a** Radiolucent lesions at apices of three mandibular incisors. **b** Mineralized masses at apices of mandibular incisors

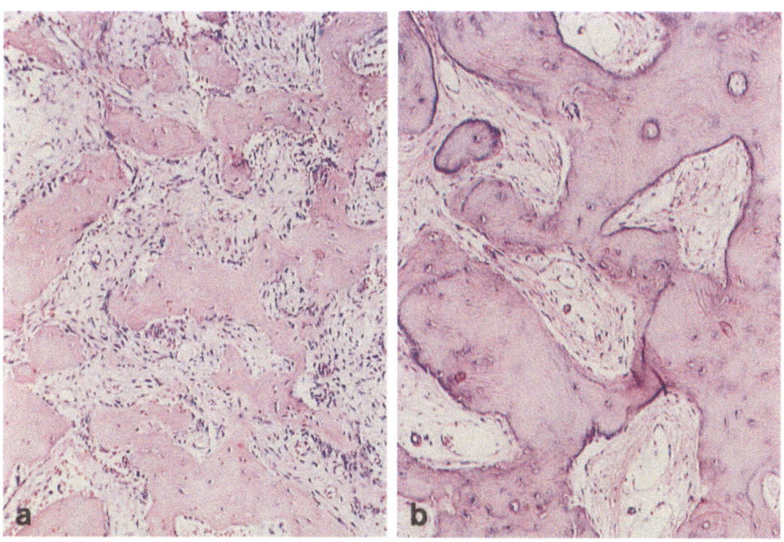


**Fig. 86 a, b.** *Periapical cemental dysplasia.* **a** Metaplastic bone. ×80. **b** Cementum-like tissue. ×80

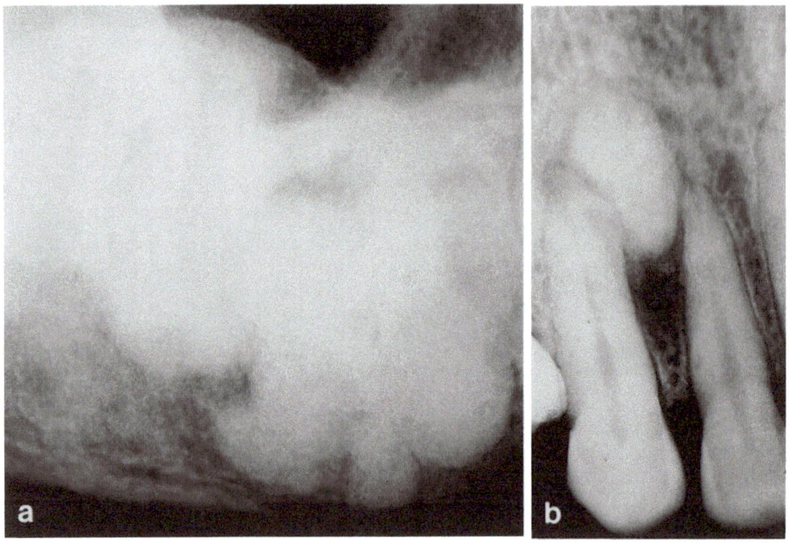

**Fig. 87 a, b.** *Florid cemento-osseous dysplasia.* **a** Lobulated dense mass in maxillary molar region. **b** Same patient; smaller mass in incisor/canine region

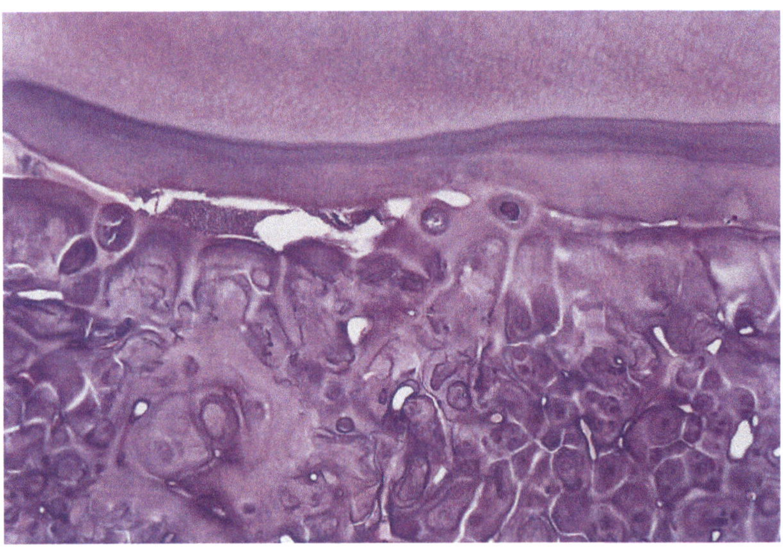

**Fig. 88.** *Florid cemento-osseous dysplasia.* Basophilic cementum-like material partly fused to root surface. ×30

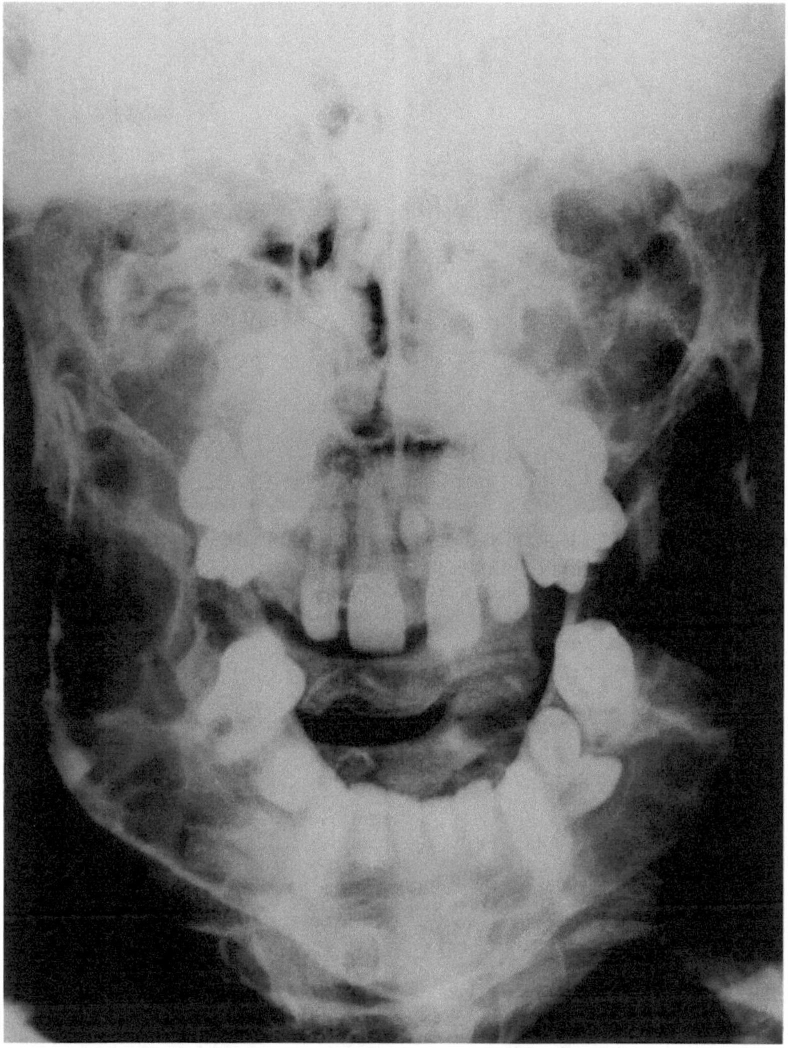

**Fig. 89.** *Cherubism.* All four quadrants of the jaws are affected

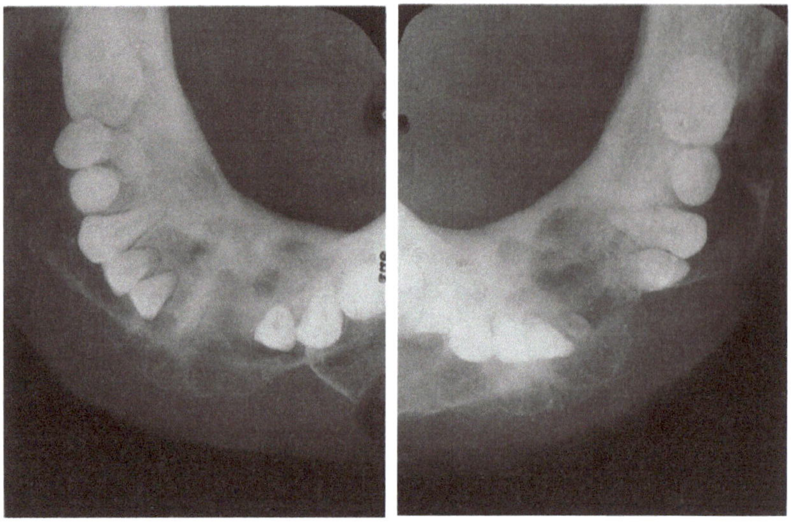

**Fig. 90.** *Cherubism.* Occlusal radiographs of mandible. Multilocular 'cystic' appearance and expansion of bone

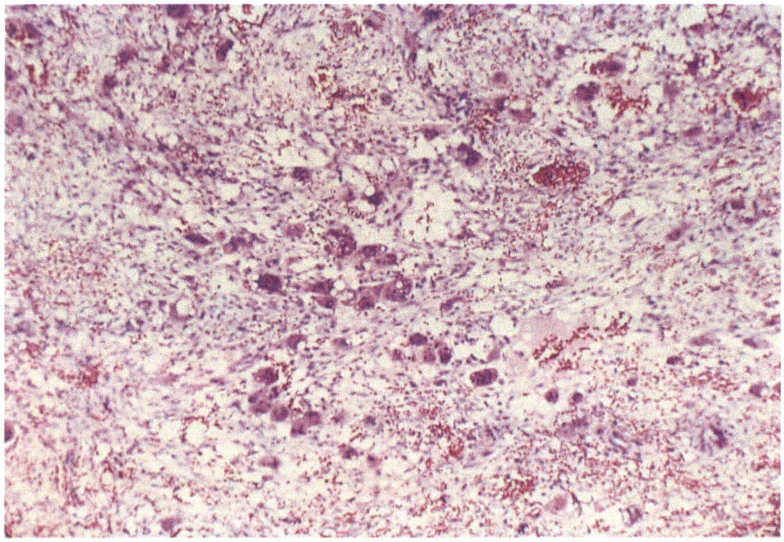

**Fig. 91.** *Cherubism.* ×80

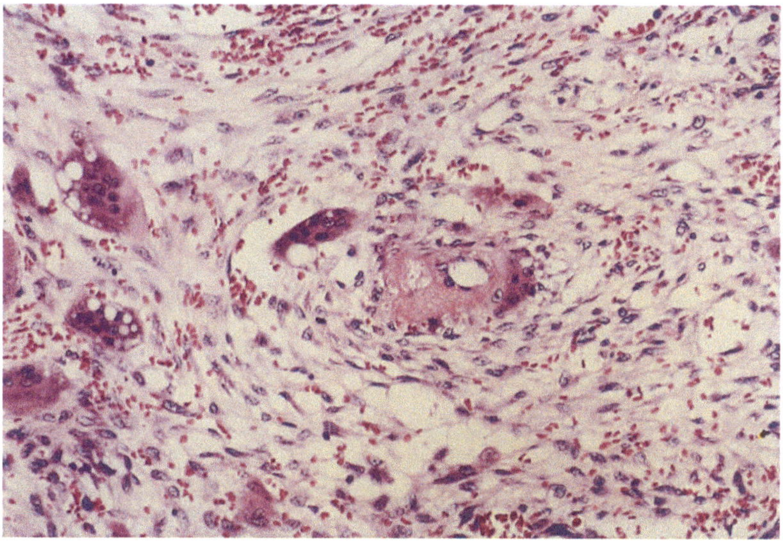

**Fig. 92.** *Cherubism.* Perivascular cuff. ×200

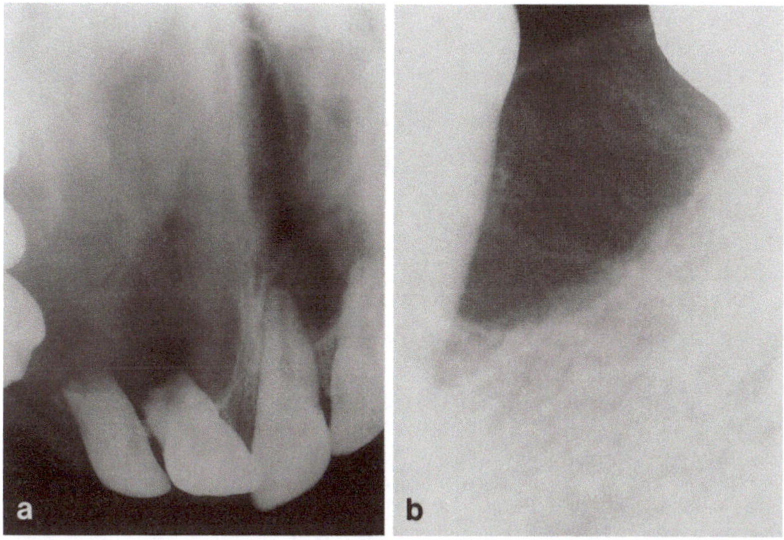


**Fig. 93 a, b.** *Giant cell granuloma.* **a** Maxilla; loculated radiolucency. **b** Mandible; slender bony septa within lesion

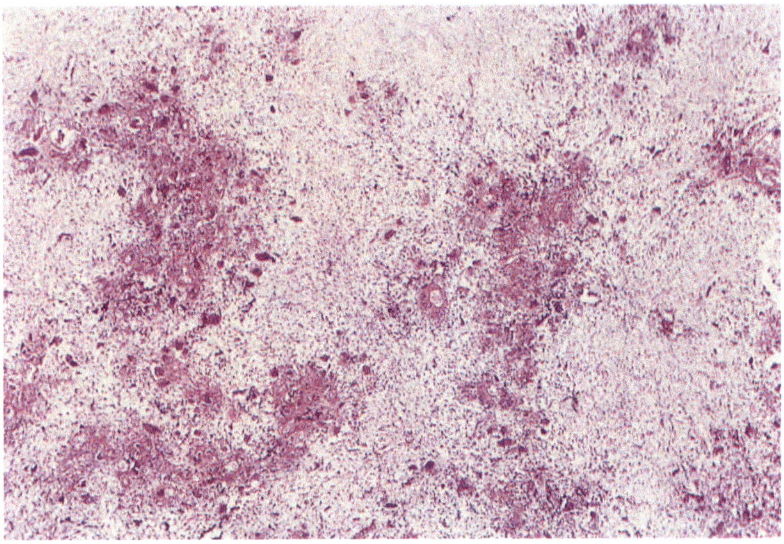

**Fig. 94.** *Giant cell granuloma.* Focal giant cell aggregation. ×32

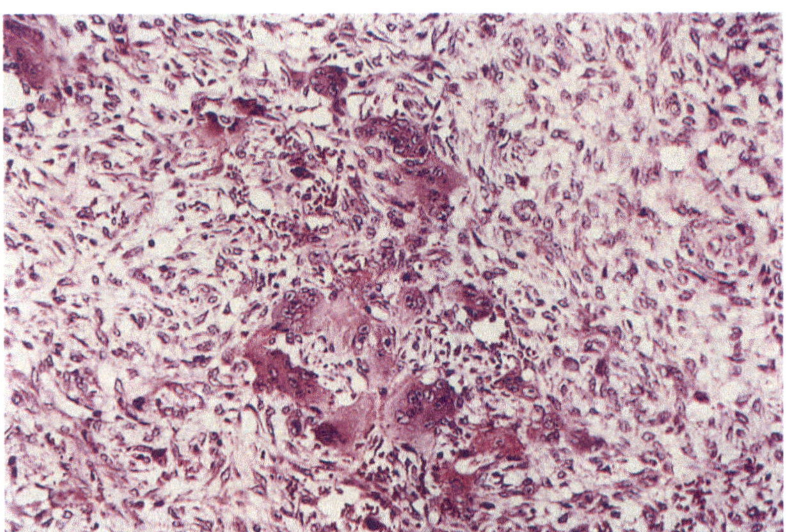

**Fig. 95.** *Giant cell granuloma.* Giant cell focus in loose-textured fibrous tissue. ×200

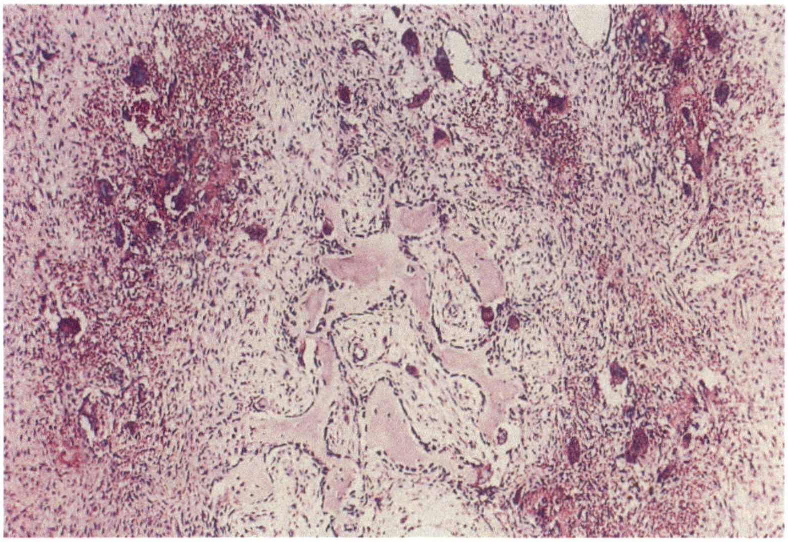

**Fig. 96.** *Giant cell granuloma.* New bone formed within the lesion. ×80

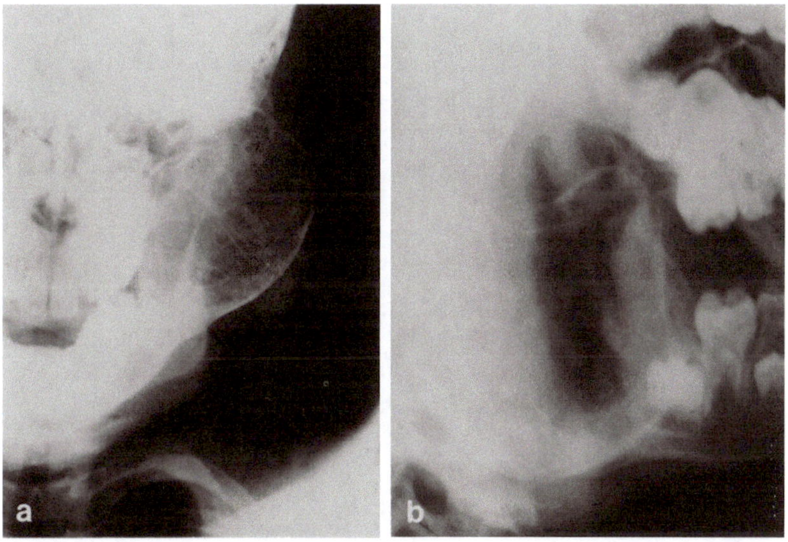


**Fig. 97 a, b.** *Aneurysmal bone cyst,* mandible

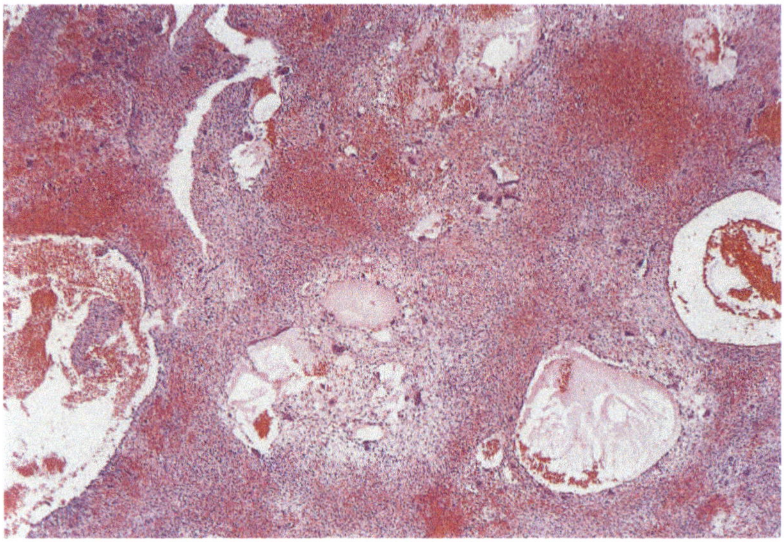

**Fig. 98.** *Aneurysmal bone cyst.* Multiple blood-filled spaces. ×25

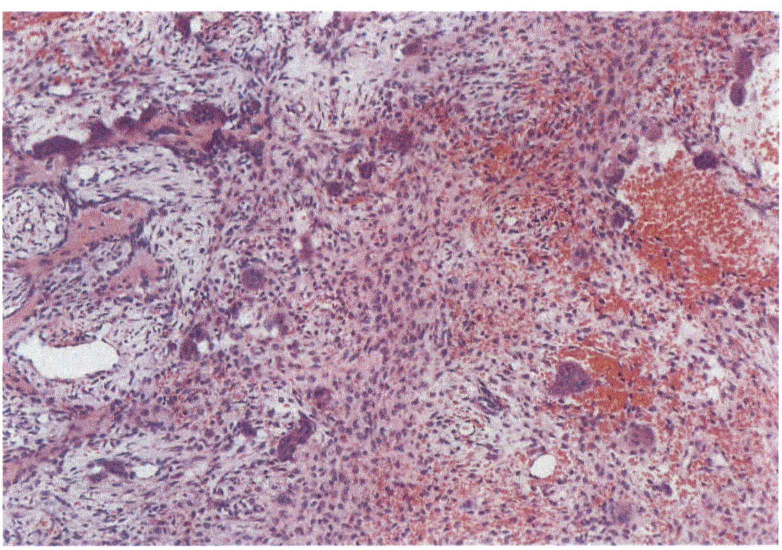

**Fig. 99.** *Aneurysmal bone cyst.* ×90

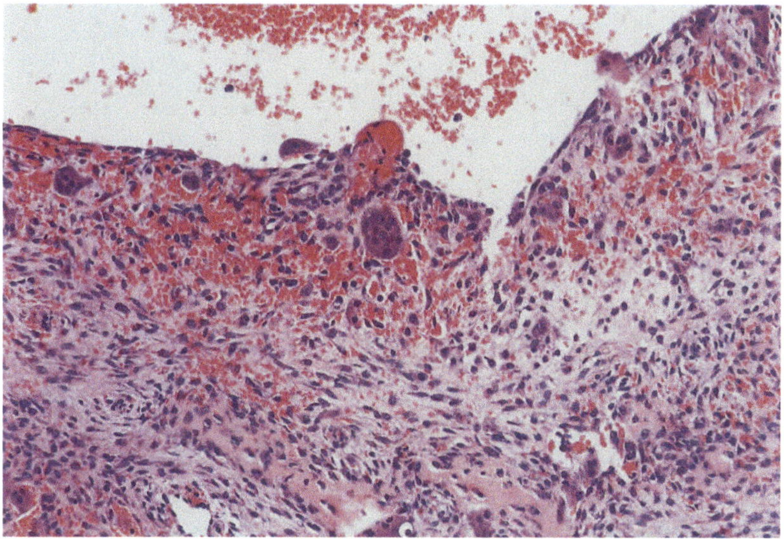

**Fig. 100.** *Aneurysmal bone cyst.* Margin of cavernous space. × 150

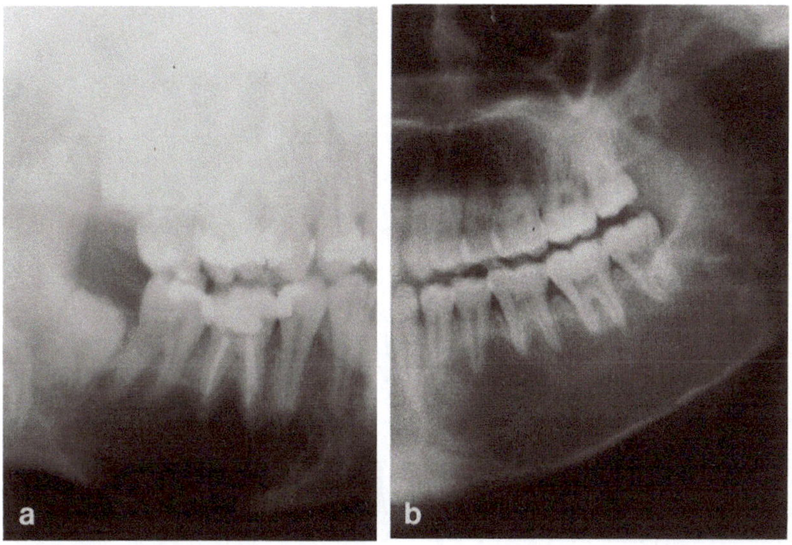


**Fig. 101 a, b.** *Solitary bone cysts.* Typical scalloped margins between roots of teeth

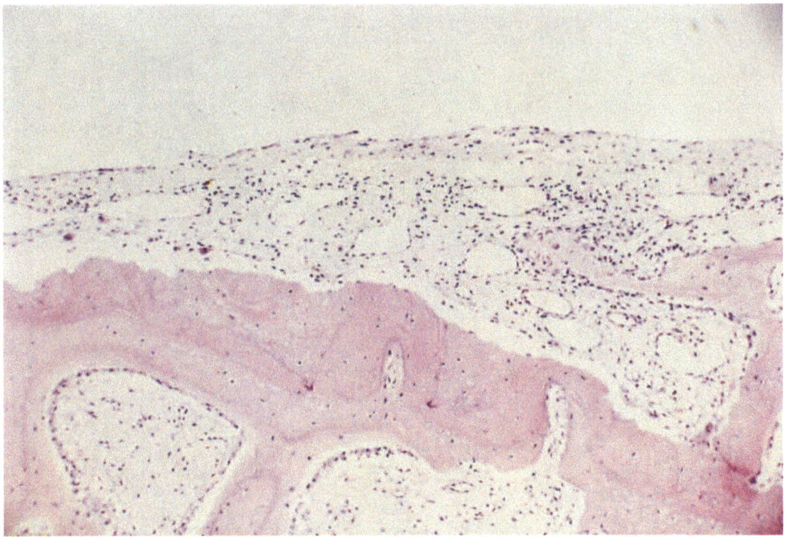

**Fig. 102.** *Solitary bone cyst.* Loose-textured cyst wall and adjacent bone. ×80

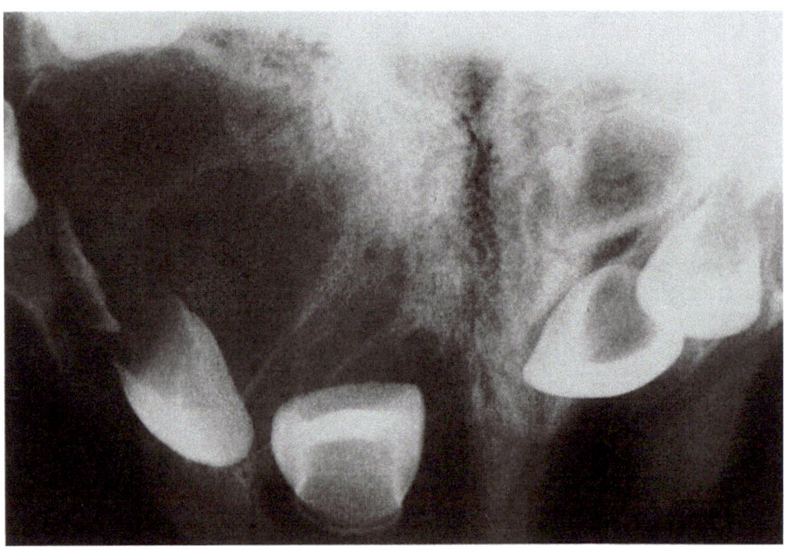

**Fig. 103.** *Melanotic neuroectodermal tumour of infancy,* maxilla. Developing teeth are displaced

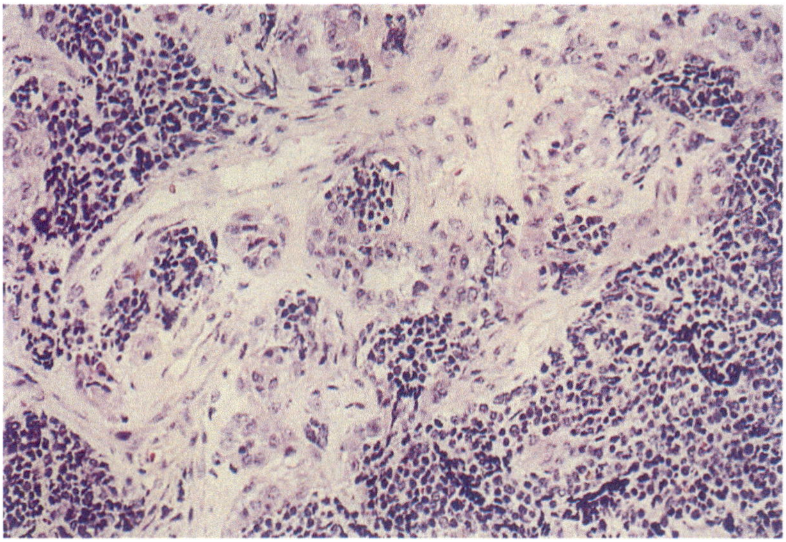

**Fig. 104.** *Melanotic neuroectodermal tumour of infancy.* Small, round, darkly staining cells and larger pale cells. ×200

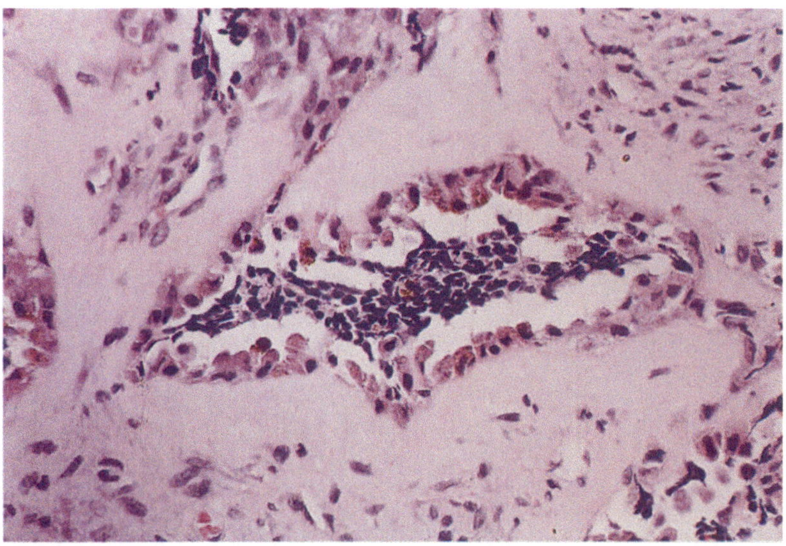

**Fig. 105.** *Melanotic neuroectodermal tumour of infancy.* Strand of pale cells with lymphocyte-like cells within cleft. ×320

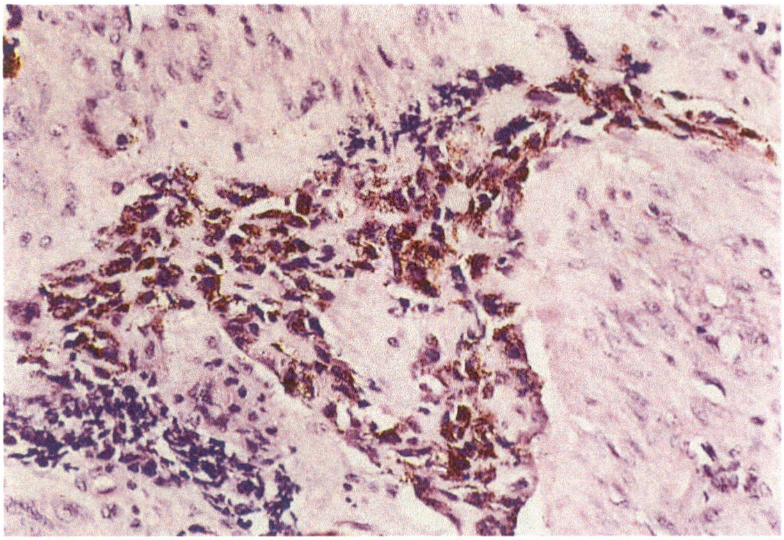

**Fig. 106.** *Melanotic neuroectodermal tumour of infancy.* Melanin in epithelium-like cells. ×320

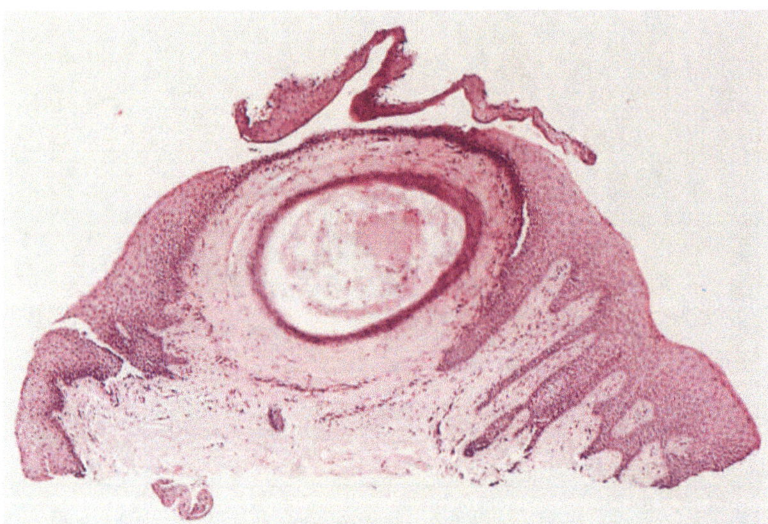

**Fig. 107.** *Gingival cyst of infant.* Keratin-filled cyst in oral mucosa. ×16

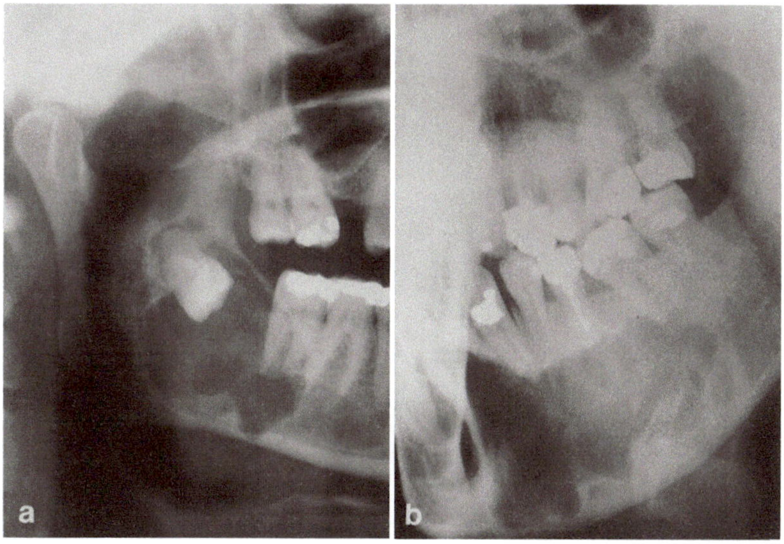


**Fig. 108 a, b.** *Odontogenic keratocysts,* mandible. Both examples show scalloped borders

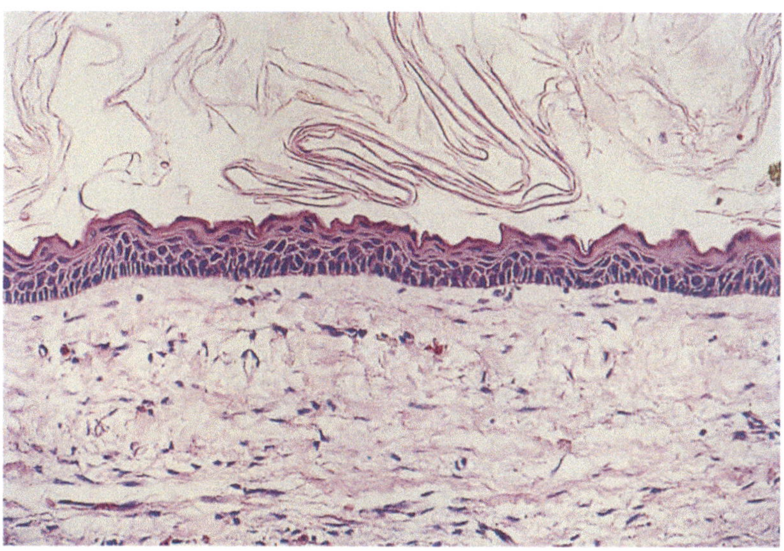

**Fig. 109.** *Odontogenic keratocyst.* Thin parakeratinized epithelium. ×200

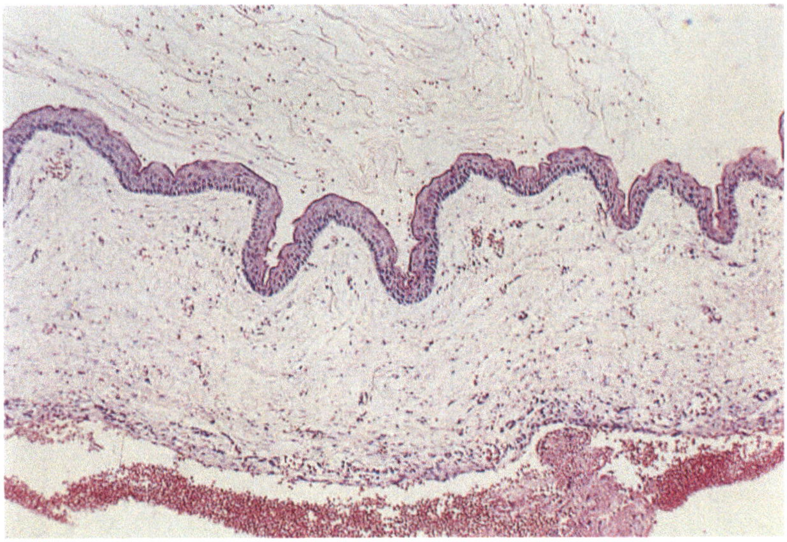

**Fig. 110.** *Odontogenic keratocyst.* Corrugated appearance of cyst wall. ×80

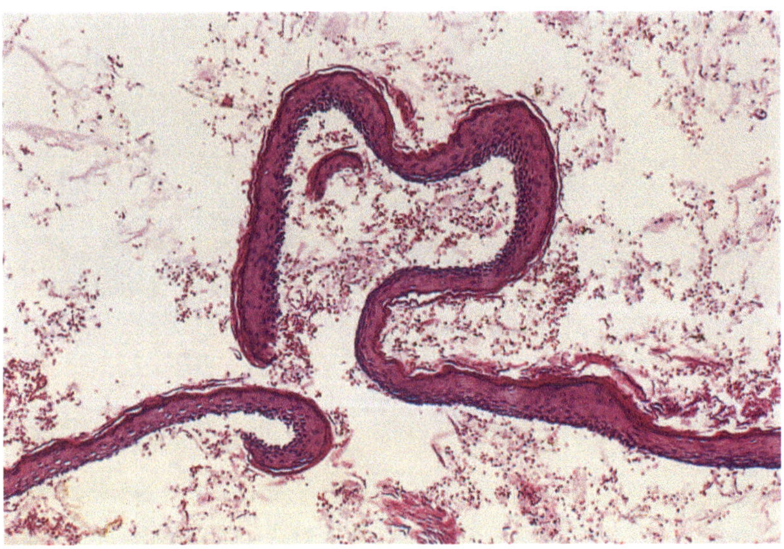

**Fig. 111.** *Odontogenic keratocyst.* Detached epithelial lining. ×80

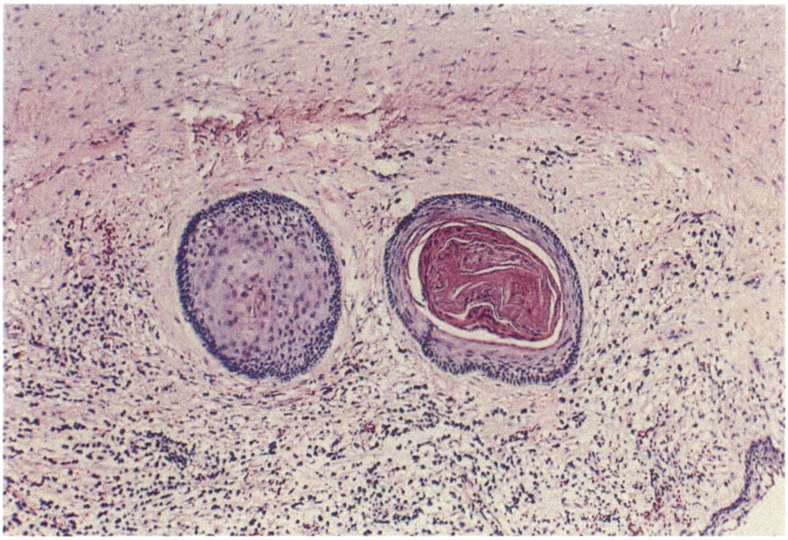

**Fig. 112.** *Odontogenic keratocyst.* Epithelial islands or daughter cysts in wall of main cyst. ×80

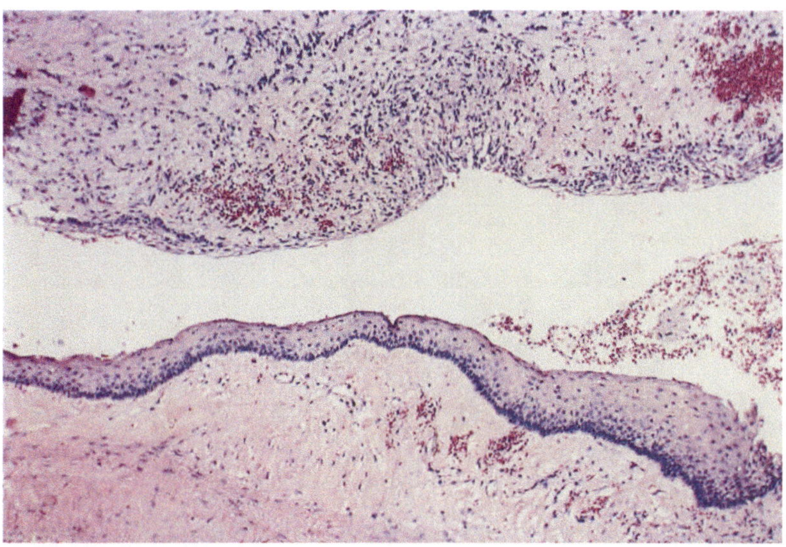

**Fig. 113.** *Odontogenic keratocyst.* Two sides of same cyst showing loss of keratinization in areas of inflammation. ×80

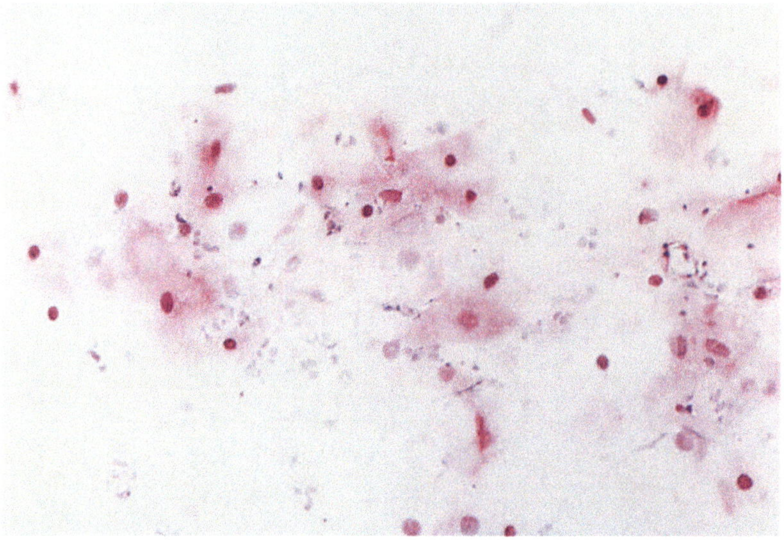

**Fig. 114.** *Odontogenic keratocyst.* Smear from aspirated cyst contents. Parakeratinized squames with ill-defined margins. ×320

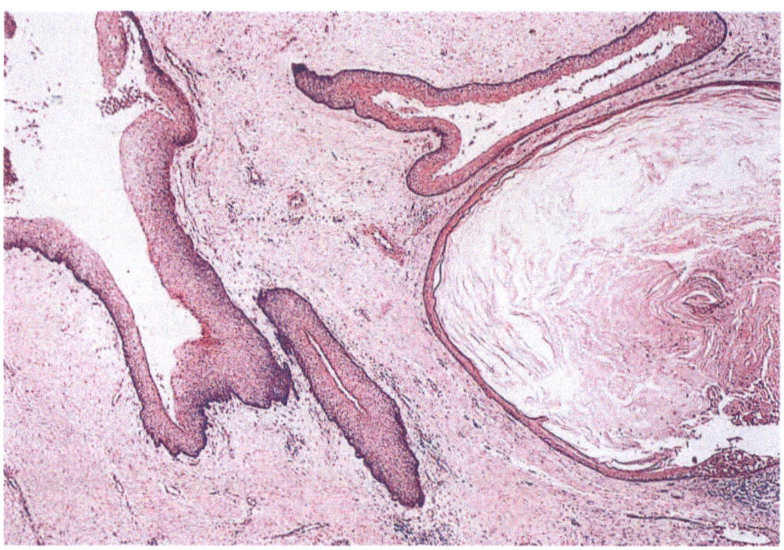

**Fig. 115.** *Odontogenic keratocyst.* Multiple keratocysts in patient with multiple naevoid basal cell carcinoma jaw cyst syndrome. ×32

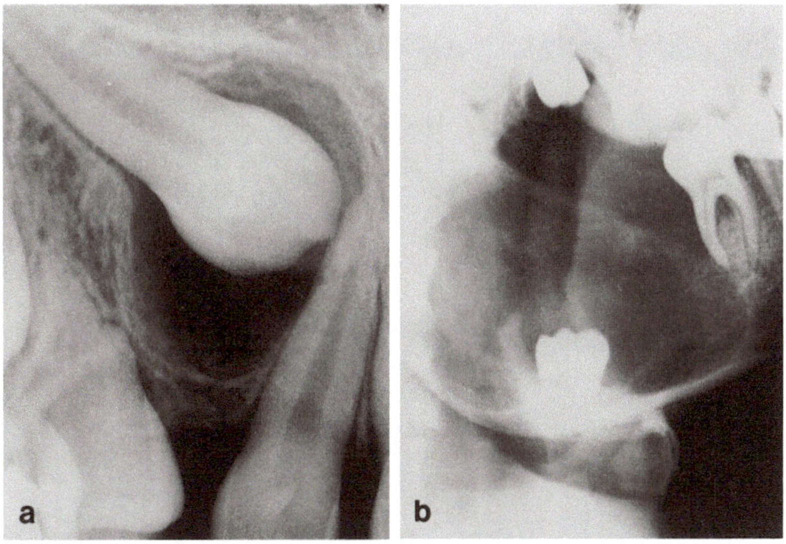


**Fig. 116 a, b.** *Dentigerous cysts.* **a** Maxillary lesion; typical enclosure of crown of tooth. **b** Large mandibular cyst

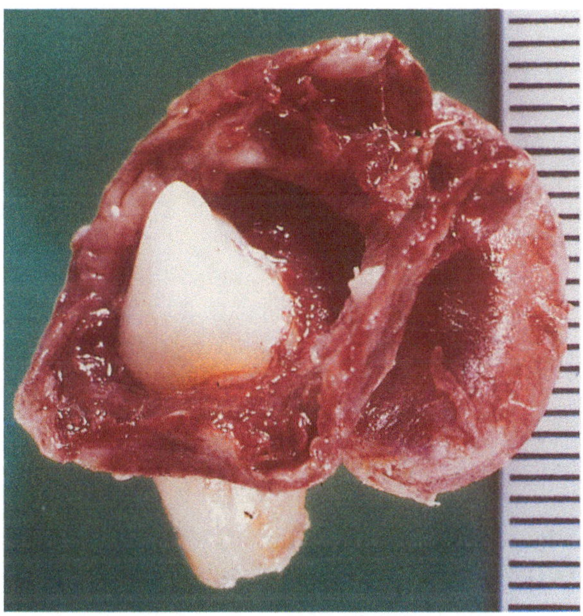

**Fig. 117.** *Dentigerous cyst.* Cyst opened to show relationship to crown of tooth

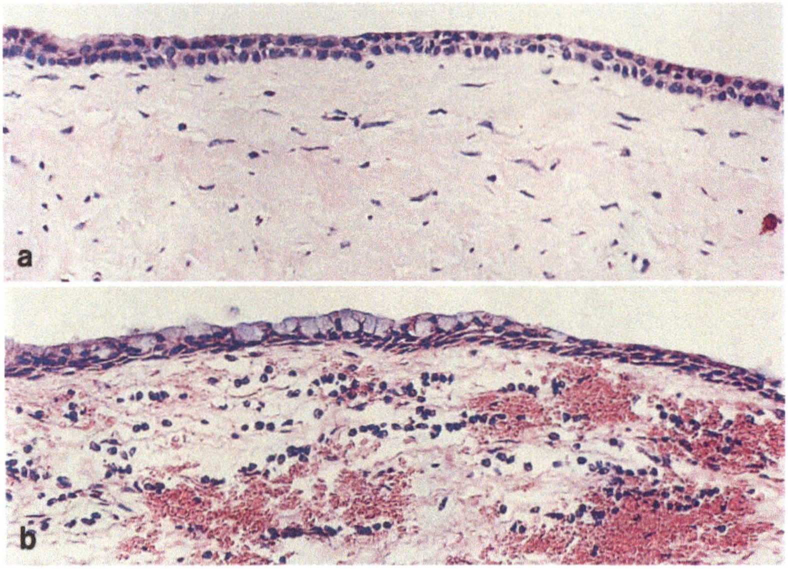


**Fig. 118 a, b.** *Dentigerous cyst.* **a** Thin epithelial lining. ×200. **b** Lining includes mucous cells. ×255

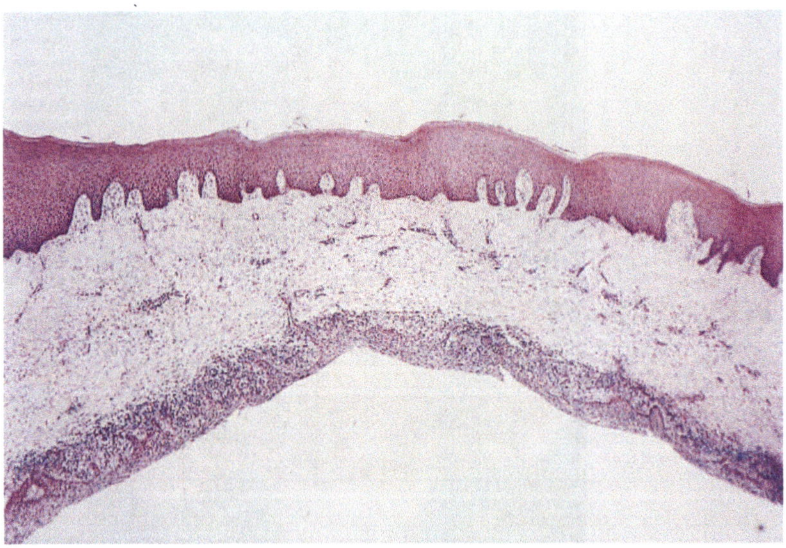

**Fig. 119.** *Eruption cyst.* Cyst lining beneath oral mucosa. ×32

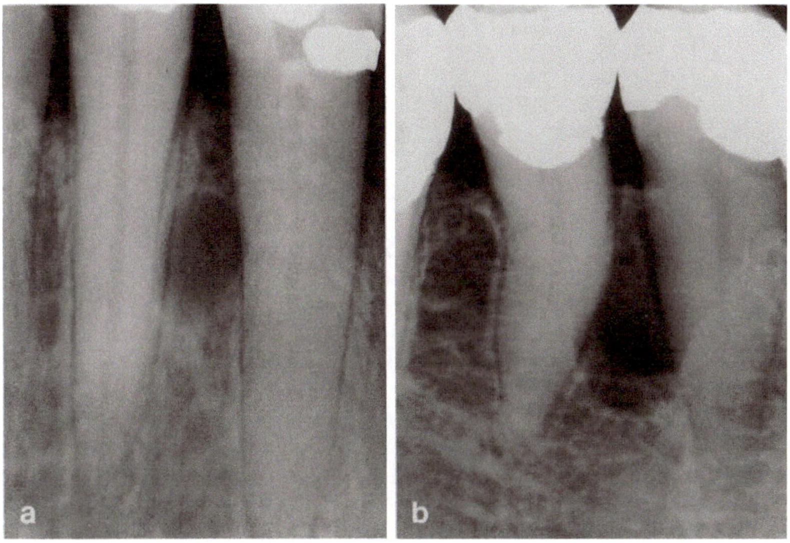


**Fig. 120 a, b.** *Lateral periodontal cysts*

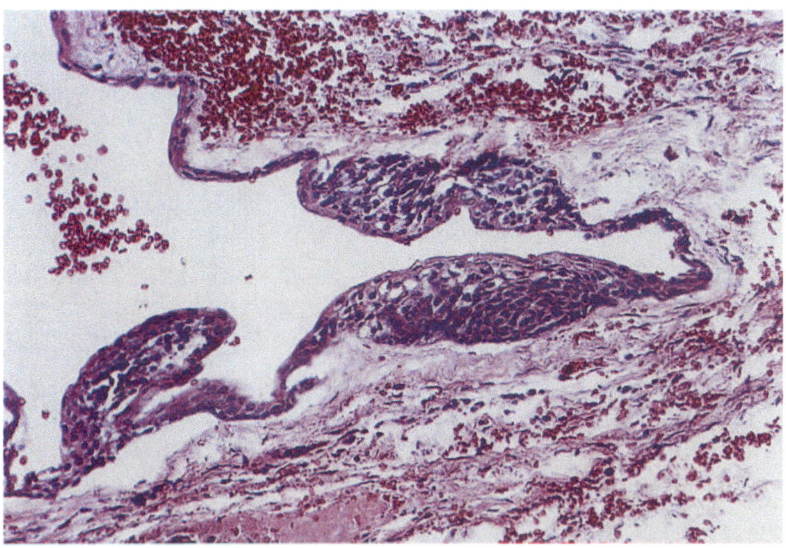

**Fig. 121.** *Lateral periodontal cyst.* Characteristic plaques in epithelial lining. ×200

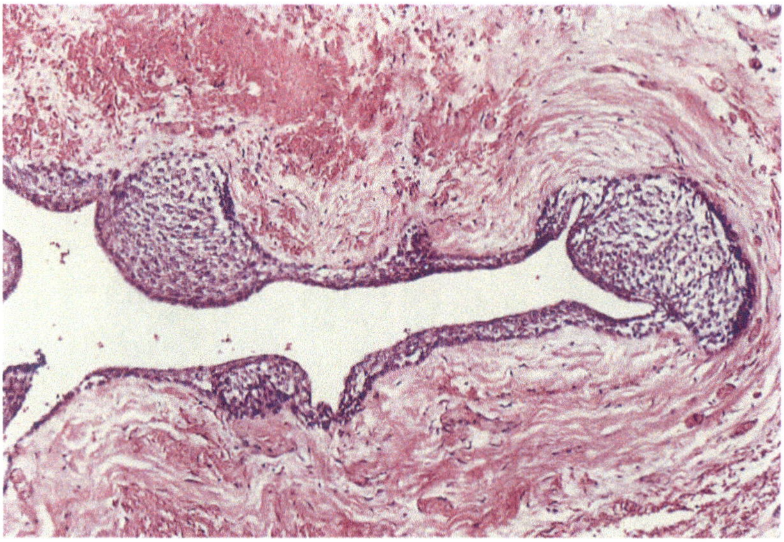

**Fig. 122.** *Lateral periodontal cyst.* Plaques partly composed of clear cells. ×100

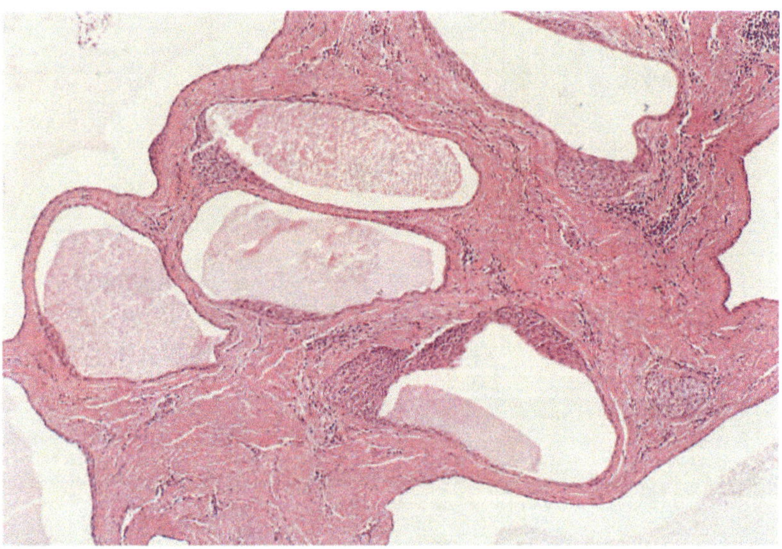

**Fig. 123.** *Botryoid odontogenic cyst.* ×50

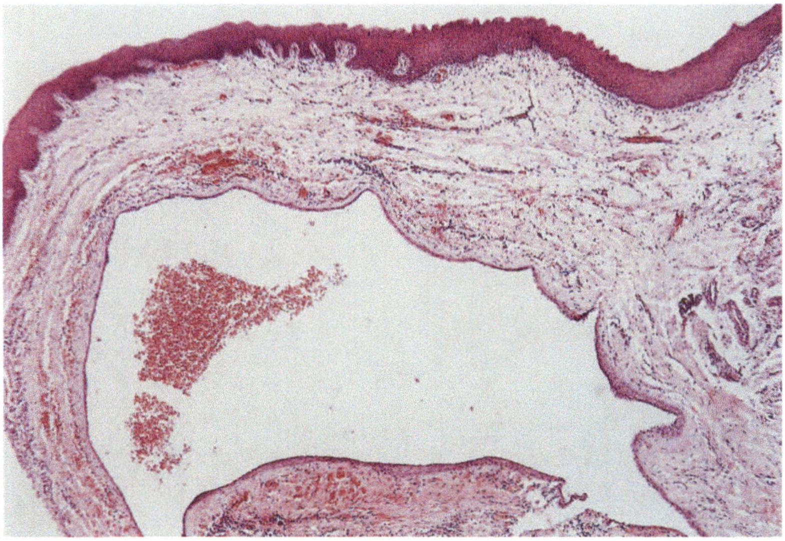

**Fig. 124.** *Gingival cyst of adult.* ×40

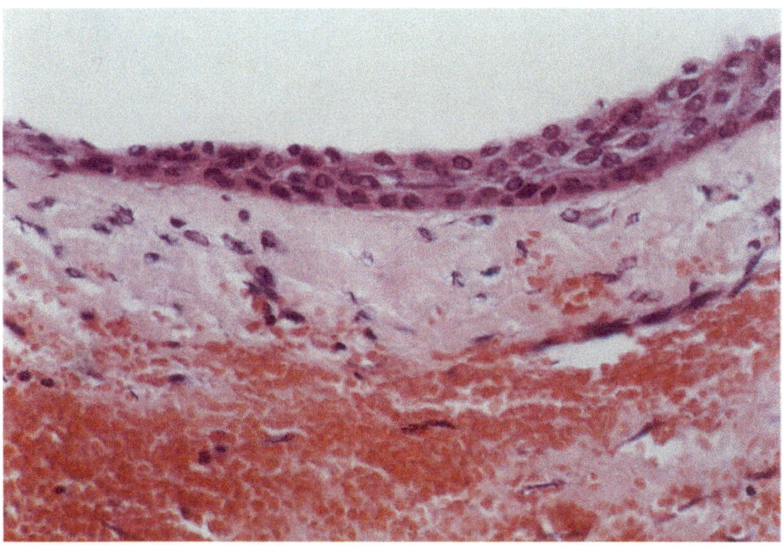

**Fig. 125.** *Gingival cyst of adult.* ×320

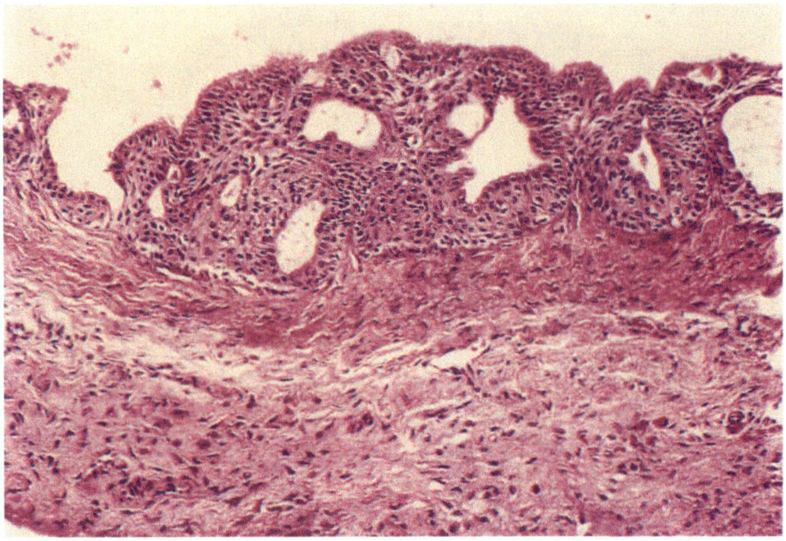

**Fig. 126.** *Glandular odontogenic cyst.* Multiple cyst-like spaces or crypts within lining epithelium. × 160

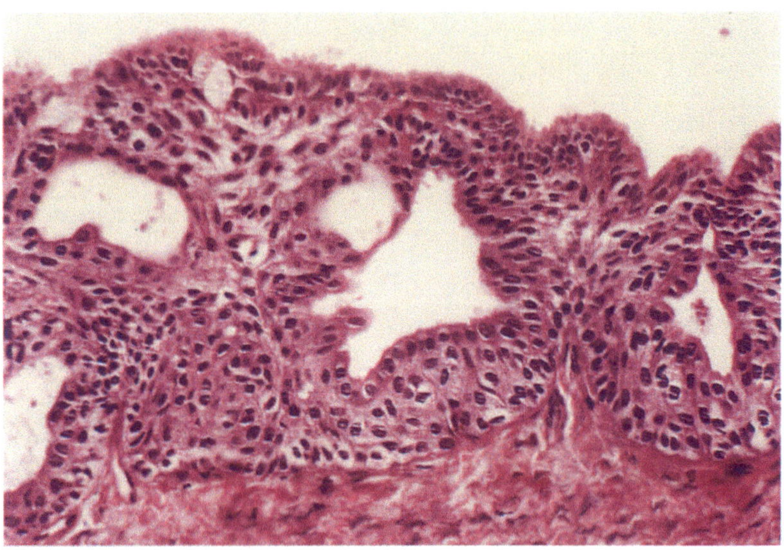

**Fig. 127.** *Glandular odontogenic cyst.* Cuboidal cells at surface and bordering spaces within epithelial cyst lining. × 320

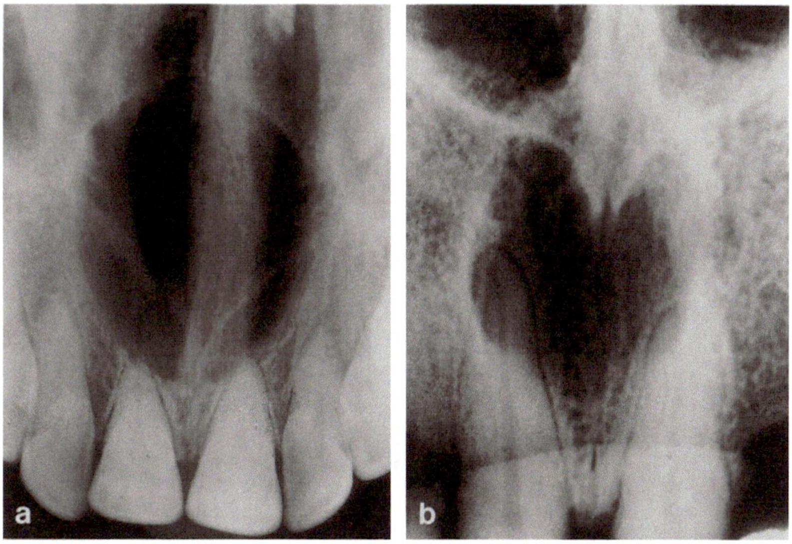


**Fig. 128 a, b.** *Nasopalatine duct cysts*

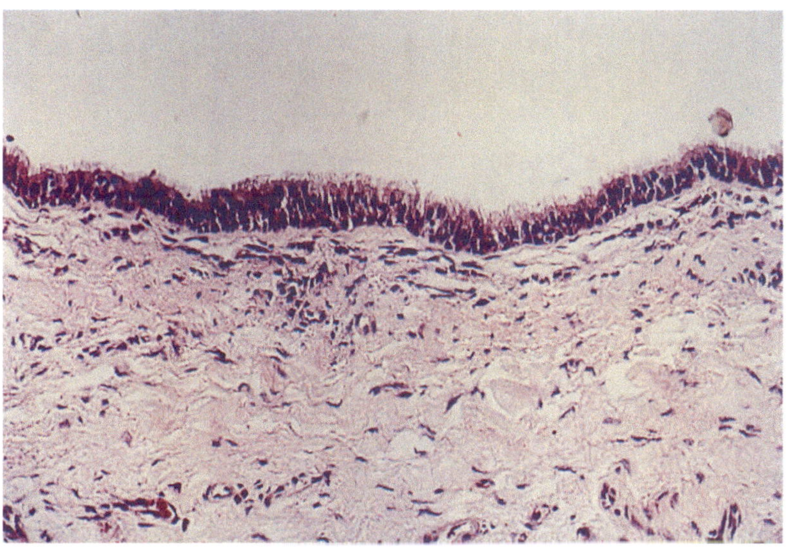

**Fig. 129.** *Nasopalatine duct cyst.* Ciliated epithelium. ×200

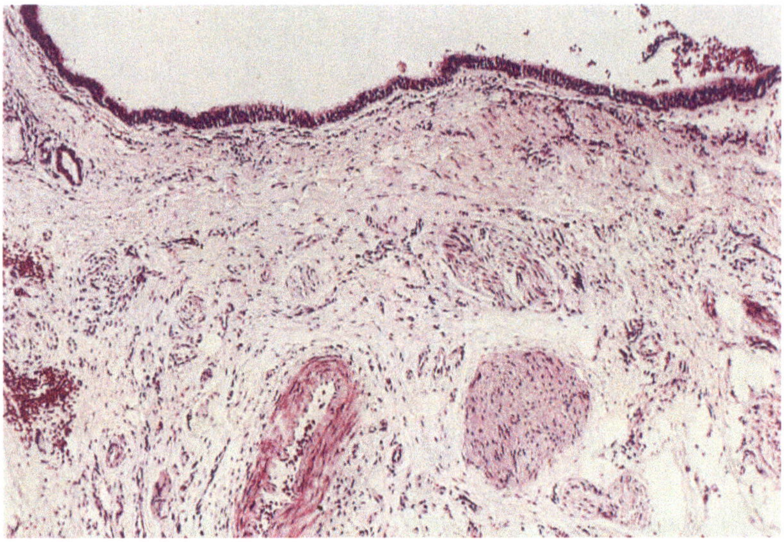

**Fig. 130.** *Nasopalatine duct cyst.* Cyst wall includes large nerve bundles, vessels and adipose tissue. ×80

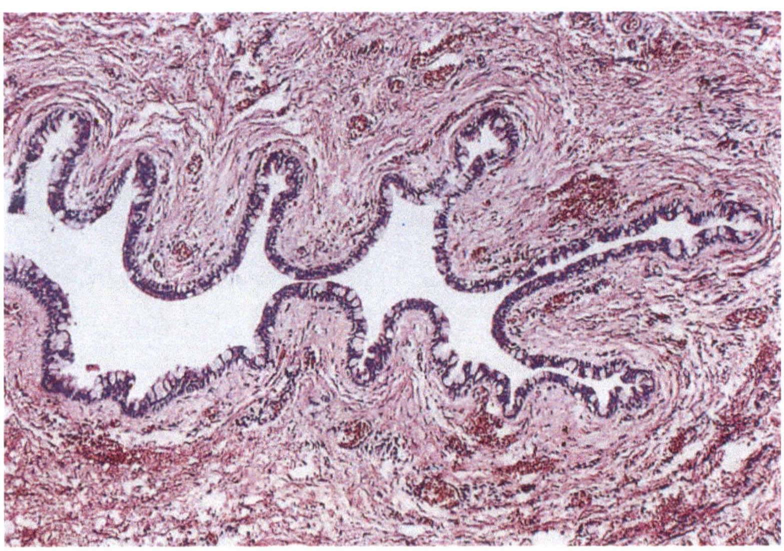

**Fig. 131.** *Nasolabial cyst.* Corrugated lining and abundant mucous cells. ×80

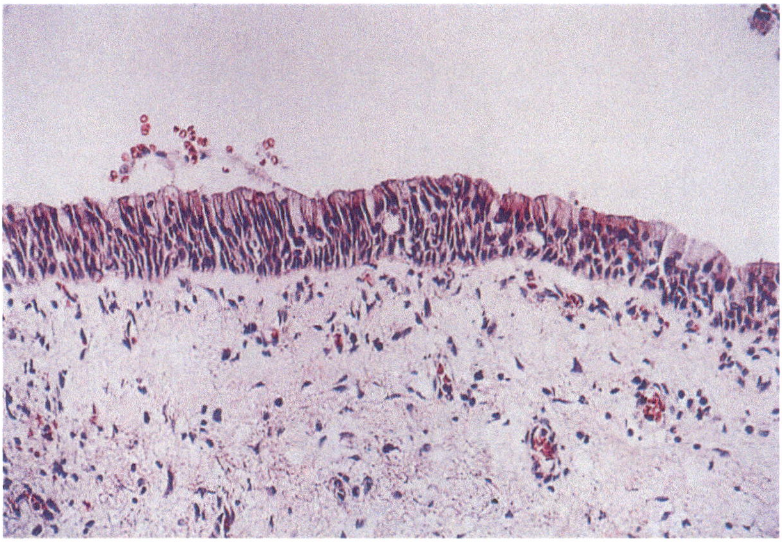

**Fig. 132.** *Nasolabial cyst.* Pseudostratified columnar epithelium. ×200

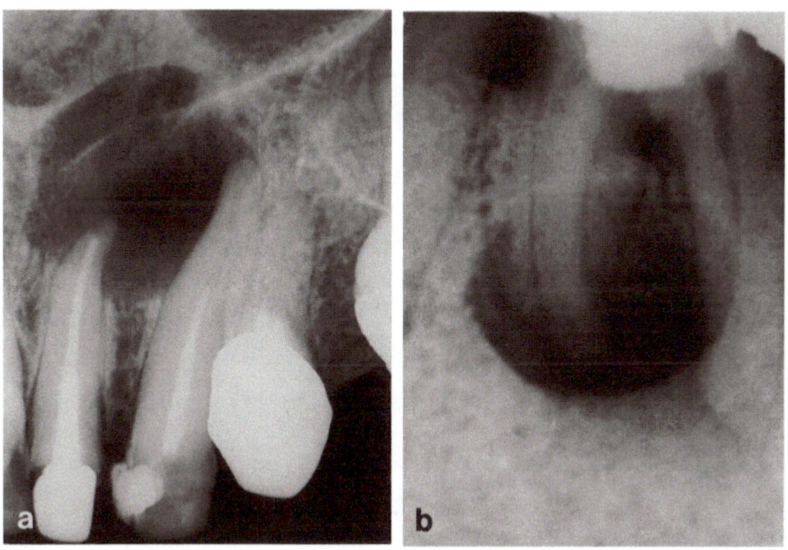

**Fig. 133 a, b.** *Radicular cyst.* **a** From root-filled maxillary incisor. **b** From mandibular molar

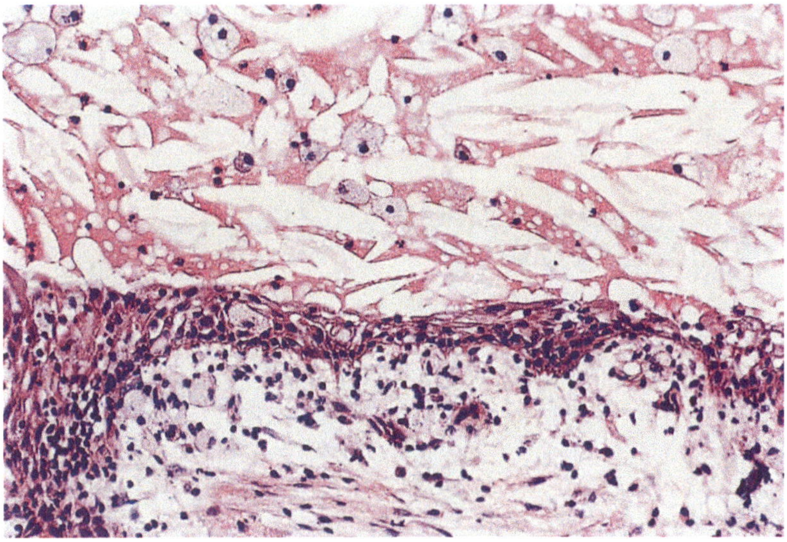

**Fig. 134.** *Radicular cyst.* Non-keratinized stratified lining. ×200

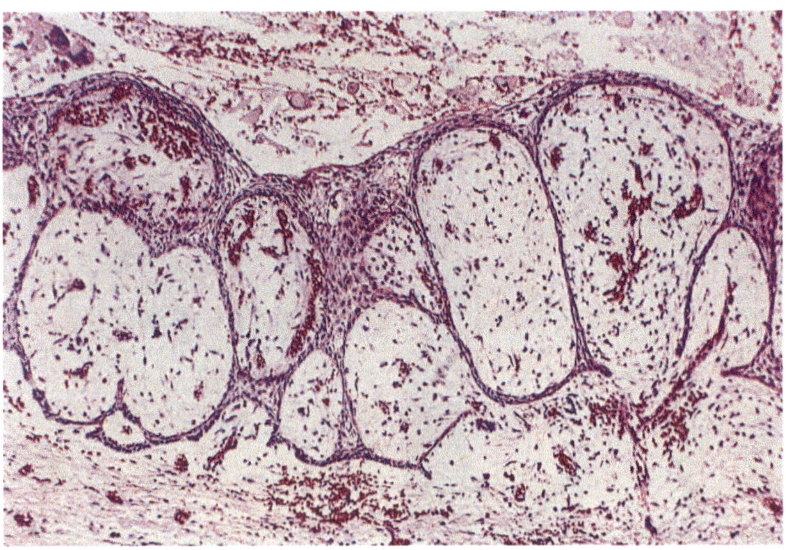

**Fig. 135.** *Radicular cyst.* ×80

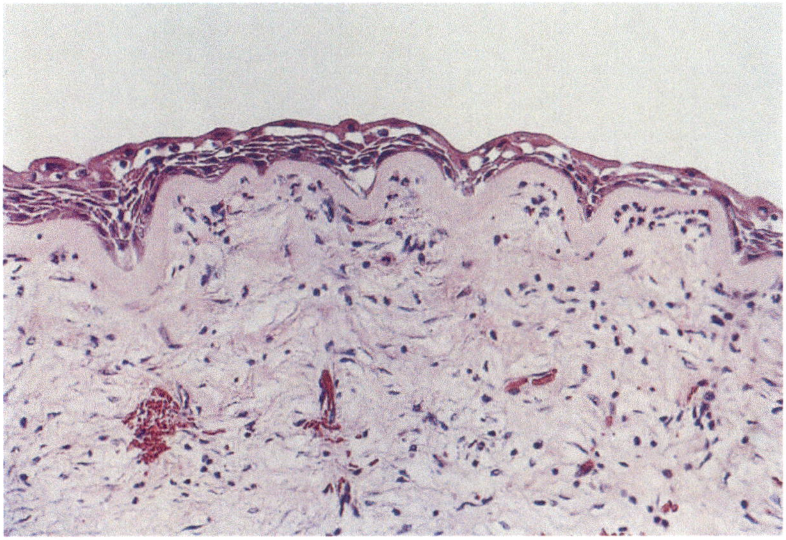

**Fig. 136.** *Radicular cyst.* Juxtaepithelial hyalinization. ×200

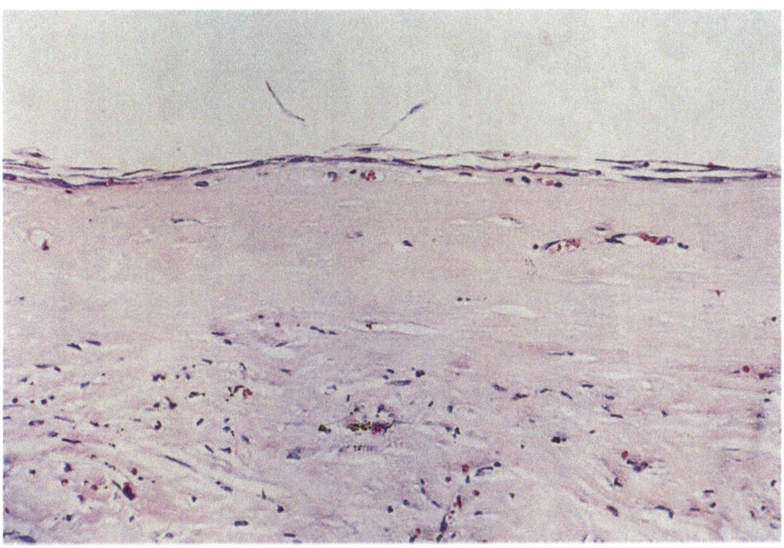

**Fig. 137.** *Radicular cyst.* Extensive hyalinization of fibrous wall and tenuous epithelial lining. ×200

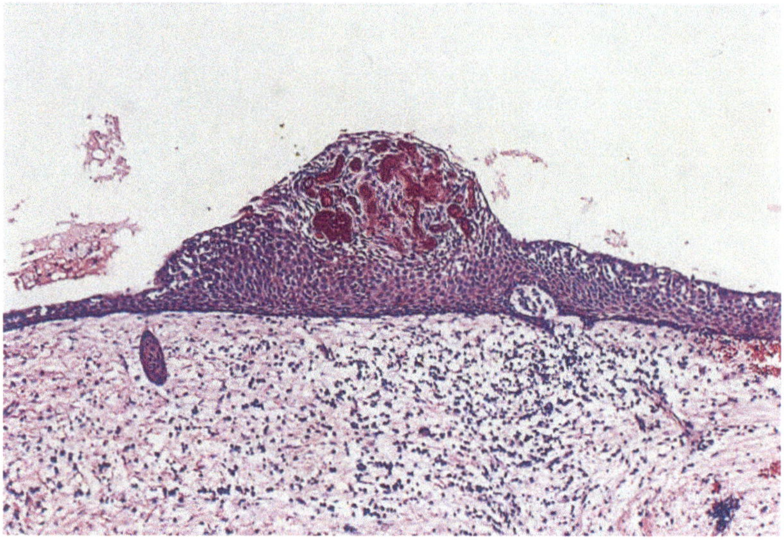

**Fig. 138.** *Radicular cyst.* Hyaline bodies in epithelium. ×12

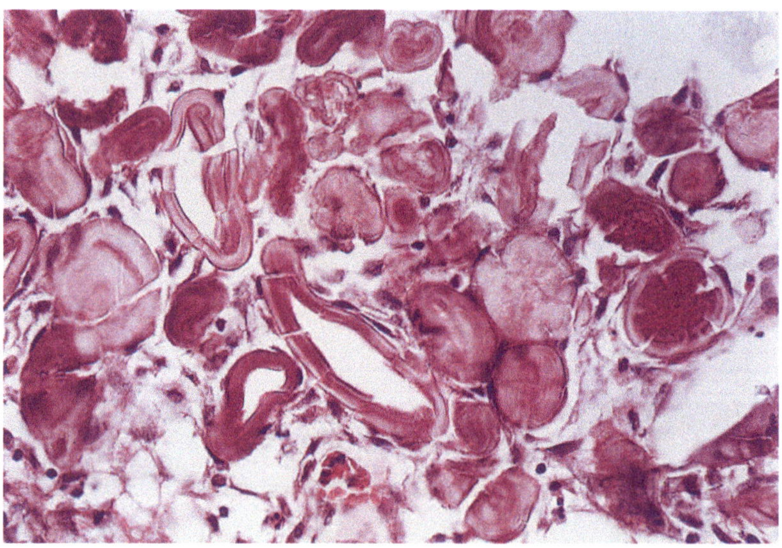

**Fig. 139.** *Radicular cyst.* Hyaline bodies. ×320

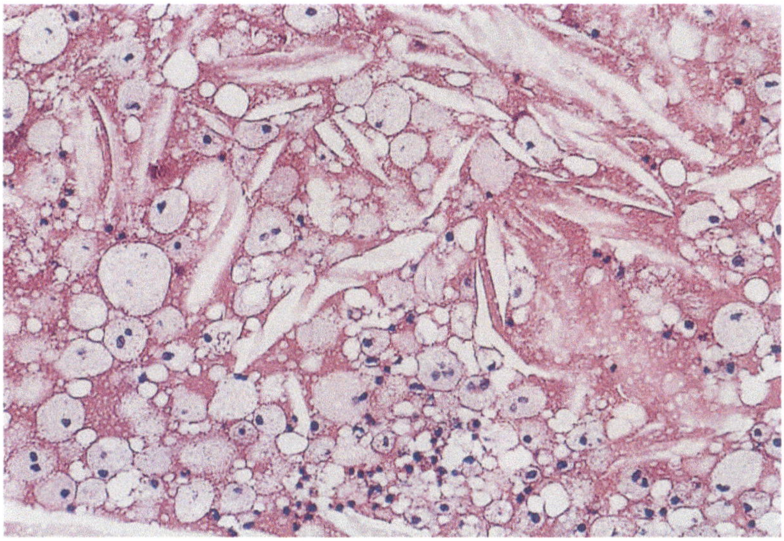

**Fig. 140.** *Radicular cyst.* Foam cells and cholesterol crystal clefts in cyst contents. ×200

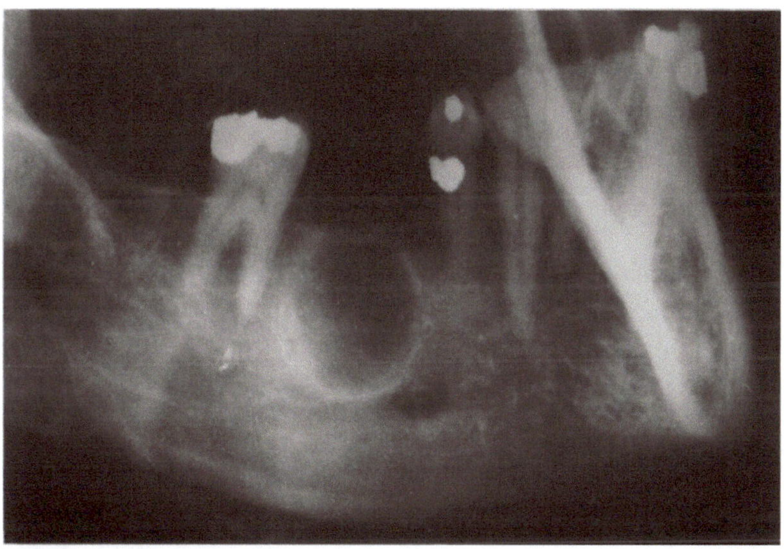

**Fig. 141.** *Residual cyst*

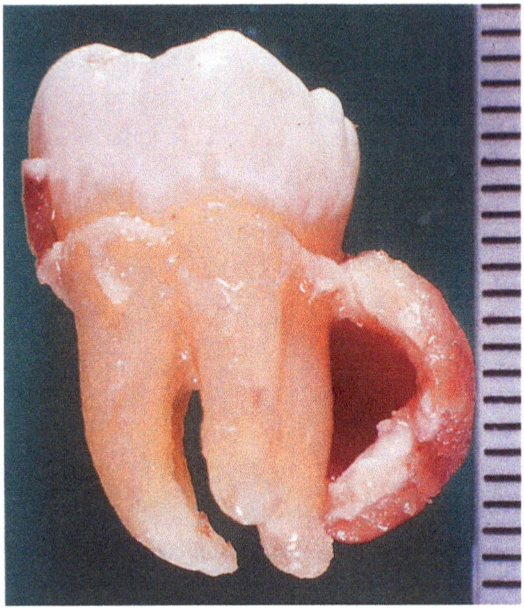

al aspect of mandibular third

*WHO International Histological Classification of Tumours*
Kramer/Pindborg/Shear:
Histological Typing of Odontogenic Tumours, 2nd edn.

**35 mm Transparencies**

A set of 159 slides (121 in colour, 38 in monochrome), corresponding to the illustrations in this book, is available from the American Registry of Pathology. To order these *slides,* send the following information to:

American Registry of Pathology
14th Street and Alaska Ave. NW
Washington, DC 20306 USA

Please send me:

________ set(s) of 35 mm slides of Histological Typing of Odontogenic Tumours at $ 100.00 per set.
For Air Mail outside of North America add $ 10.00.

Total cost: $ ______.00

Name ________________________________________

Address ______________________________________

______________________________________________

______________________________________________

Date ________________ Signature ________________

☐ I enclose a check/money order in US $ payable to the ARP.
☐ Please charge my credit card:
 ☐ VISA
 ☐ MasterCard

Card number __________________________________

Expiration date ________________________________

Name as it appears on credit card ______________________

Prices are subject to change without notice.

MIX
Papier aus verantwortungsvollen Quellen
Paper from responsible sources
FSC® C105338

If you have any concerns about our products,
you can contact us on
**ProductSafety@springernature.com**

In case Publisher is established outside the EU,
the EU authorized representative is:
**Springer Nature Customer Service Center GmbH**
**Europaplatz 3, 69115 Heidelberg, Germany**

Printed by Libri Plureos GmbH
in Hamburg, Germany